MW00891591

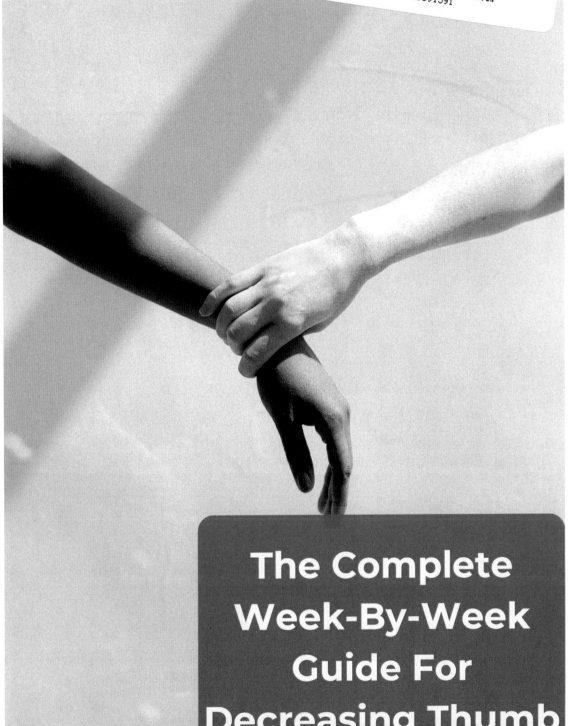

The Complete Week-By-Week Guide For Decreasing Thumb And Wrist Pain (DeQuervain's)

About Our Expert

Hi! My name is Rose and I have practiced as an Orthopedic Occupational Therapist for over 17 years. My specialty and focus is in treating injuries of the bones, muscles, nerves and ligaments of the hands, wrists, arms and shoulders. I have always loved and continue to love what I do. It is a special privilege to help individuals regain function in their hands, wrists, arms and shoulders so they can return back to living the life they want!

I started my company because I wanted (and still want to!) to support and serve individuals in their recovery from hand, wrist, arm and shoulder injury and pain. I understand how much these injuries can affect so many areas of our life including, and most importantly, our identity!

So I made this guide to make it infinitely easier for you to know what to do about your hand and wrist pain! It is filled with the therapeutic exercises, recommendations and education I have provided to thousands of past patients/clients.

Good luck and I'm here if you need me! I look forward to hearing about your recovery!

With so love and support,

Rose

Orthopedic Occupational Therapist and
Certified Hand Therapist
Owner First The Moms

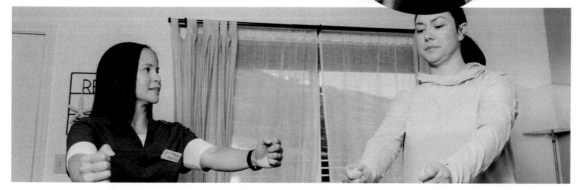

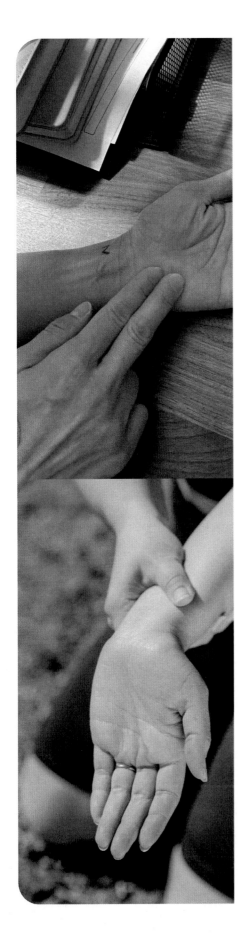

About This Guide

I designed this starter guide, like I said, to make it so much easier for you to begin to know what to do about your hand and wrist pain.

Because we are just too busy to have caring for ourselves be hard. Solutions must not only help the problem, but they must be easy to find, clear, straightforward and easy to navigate.

And this is what I kept at the forefront of my mind in designing this guide.

Filled with the therapeutic program I provide to my clients during the acute stage of their injury and pain, our guide is tells you what you should be doing at the beginning of your recovery. You never have to think about what you should be doing at any one moment.

Because when we make getting better easier than we have a better chance for success.

So thank you for purchasing this guide! Thank you for allowing me a front row seat in your journey!

For You

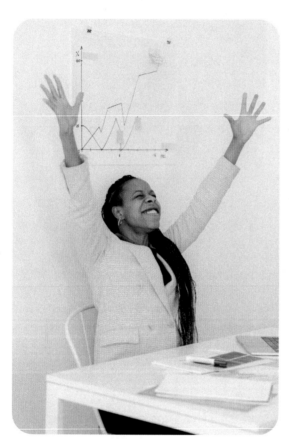

Before you start this guide and start this journey of recovery, I wanted to say bravo! Bravo to you for choosing your health, your happiness, but, most especially, for choosing YOU!! It's never easy to put your health first when life is so busy, but I am so glad you made this decision to start!

So first thing, as you are moving through the guide try and remember your why (why did you start this?). Because as you continue you will hit fatigue, you will feel overwhelmed, you might even want to give up. So keep your why/whys nearby. Remember who the why is. Yes, your loved ones, but more importantly, your why is living the life you want to live-with less pain!

So let's get started! And remember I'm cheering for you loudly!! I'm your biggest support! And I'm here for you anytime!!

Bravo to you!!

Disclaimer

By using this guide you are agreeing to the following terms of service/disclaimer: You understand and accept that this is not medical treatment and that First The Moms and all individuals affiliated with First The Moms are not your treating therapist/therapist. You understand and accept that performing these exercises /using recommended products/starting recommended modifications to your activities is at your own risk and First The Moms and all individuals affiliated with First The Moms will not be held liable for any injuries and/or worsening of injuries that may incur. You understand and accept that this information provided is general education and not for your specific injury. You understand and accept that performing these exercises/using recommended products/starting recommended modifications to your activities does not guarantee improvement of your injury and/or symptoms. Before starting any exercises or stretches, advisement by your physician is recommended.

Any dispute arising out of the digital material or on-demand courses created by First The Moms(the "Materials") shall be governed by the substantive laws of the State of California, without respect to its conflict of laws principles. You agree to submit to the jurisdiction of the courts located in the State of California, County of Orange, with respect to any dispute, disagreement, or cause of action related to or involving First the Moms or the Materials.

Table of Contents

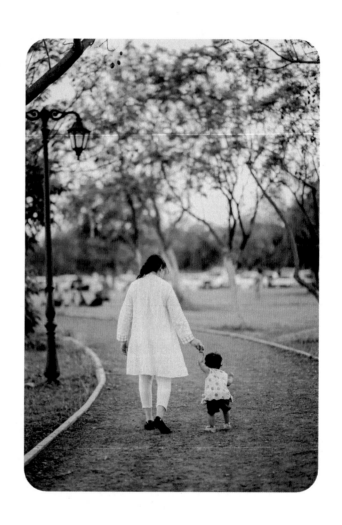

Table of Contents

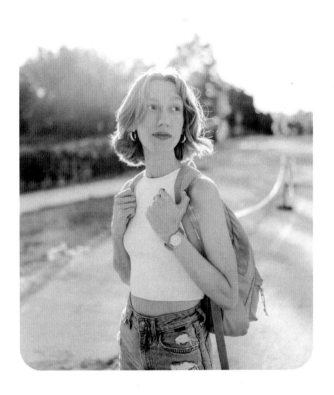

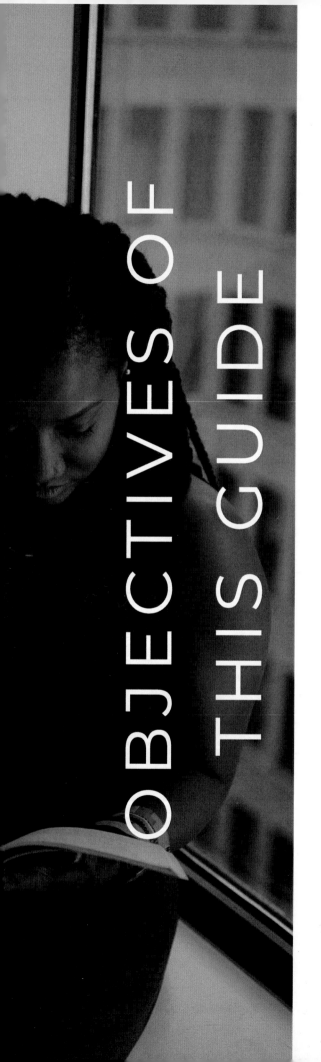

OBJECTIVES OF THIS GUIDE

1. To make it much, much easier for you to know what to do about your hand and wrist injury and pain during the beginning stage. We understand how busy you are! No more wasting valuable time trying to find out what to do!

2. To equip you with the therapeutic exercises, recommendations, and education that I have provided to thousands of clients. You will have the tools to decrease your pain now and in the future!

3. To support you in your journey to health and not just for your hands and wrists but your health overall. We want to be your biggest supporters in putting your well-being first!

About DeQuervain's

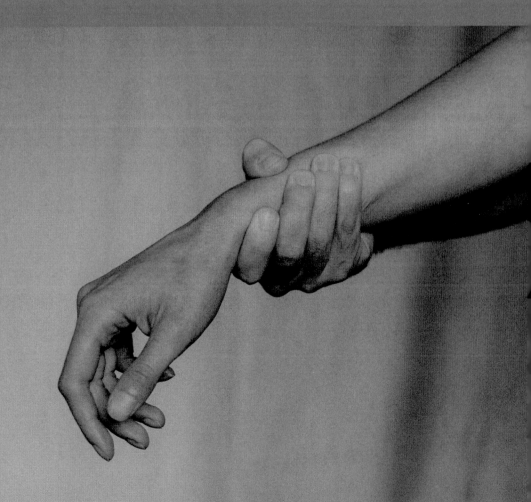

All About DeQuervain's Tenosynovitis

What is DeQuervain's?

DeQuervain's tenosynovitis (thumb and wrist pain) is a condition where, first, the tendon sheaths (the tunnels that surround the tendons) become thickened and narrow(due to inflammation or possibly degenerative changes). This then can causes constriction and friction to the tendons that normal glide through them easily during movement of the thumb and wrist. We then get pain with movement of the thumb and/or wrist.

The pain is usually felt at the wrist (where the thumb and wrist meet) with activities such as gripping, wrist movement and, generally, just using the hand. The pain can also be felt up the thumb and also up the forearm. If the condition is more severe you can also have pain at rest.

What causes DeQuervain's?

Though doctors don't know exactly what causes DeQuervain's they do know there are certain and conditions that leave you more vulnerable to DeQuervain's.

For instance, trauma to the wrist area where the pain is such as when an IV is placed in that area or that area getting hit. Those with certain medical conditions can be more at risk such as rheumatoid arthritis, diabetes and pregnancy.

However, often times, repetition of certain movement and activities (these movement and activities will be discussed in a bit) can put you more at risk.

All About DeQuervain's Tenosynovitis

Repetitive Movements That Can Leave You Vulnerable to DeQuervain's

a. Repetitive opening and closing your hand.

b. Repetitive movement of your hand side to side.

d. Repetitive or sustained gripping.

c. Repetitive movements of your thumb away from the palm.

e. Repetitive or sustained pinching.

I am sure you are now thinking "JUST USING YOUR HAND CAN LEAVE YOU VULNERABLE!" And I am sure that leaves you frustrated and hopeless. But it IS NOT USING YOUR HAND but more like *HOW YOU ARE USING YOUR HAND* that has left you vulnerable to injury and pain. Often times when we do our everyday activities we are using our hands for a long period and doing a motion repetitively. This leads to injury and pain!

But how do we change how we are using our hand? Well, that is what this guide is all about (And specifically week 3 of this guide! In week 3 I will teach you general understandings of how to keep your hand and wrist safe while doing activities so that you can apply them to YOUR specific activities).

My goal for you isn't to start avoiding and restricting you from certain activities. I want you to live your ENTIRE LIFE. My goal is for you to understand how to do them without leading to pain and injury!

All About DeQuervain's Tenosynovitis

What happens if I don't manage my pain and injury?

If a therapeutic program such as this is not started , eventually your symptoms will become more severe, occur more often and last longer. Tasks will become more difficult. With time, damage to the body will be permanent. At that point, therapeutic programs like this will not be effective and more invasive treatment (such as injections and surgery) will be the only option. So, as you can see, your pain and injury should not be taken lightly.

Why is this guide beneficial?

Because figuring out everything that you should be doing to prevent pain in your hand and wrist is challenging and time-consuming! And I KNOW you don't want to make your life harder by having to figure this out on your own. So why not leave it to an expert to lead you?

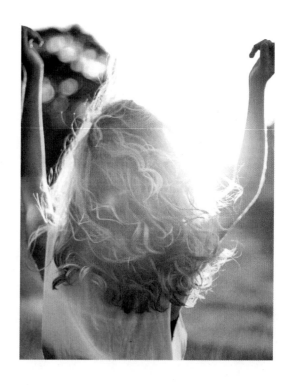

This guide was designed to be convenient, easy-to-use and organized. It not only gives you real and quality solutions to your pain, but it gives you back valuable time (not wasted on searching for answers!).

So let's get started on getting you better!!

In Case You Were Wondering...

DEQUERVAIN'S IS NOT (I REPEAT) THE SAME AS CARPAL TUNNEL SYNDROME!

These two conditions are completely different. DeQuervain's symptoms, as we discussed, are due to abnormal changes of the tendon sheaths and tendons. Carpal tunnel syndrome symptoms are due to compression of a nerve (specifically the median nerve).

DeQuervain's presents with sharp/dull pain where the thumb meets the wrist (and sometimes into the thumb and forearm) that can happen with gripping, pinching, use of the hand and with certain wrist movements. Carpal tunnel syndrome presents with, initially, numbness and tingling in the thumb, index, middle and part of the ring finger.

The only common factor that DeQuervain's and carpal tunnel syndrome have is that they are typically overuse injuries. Hence, doing a repeated movement or activity or holding a position for a long period can put the hand and wrist at risk.

Let's Get Started!

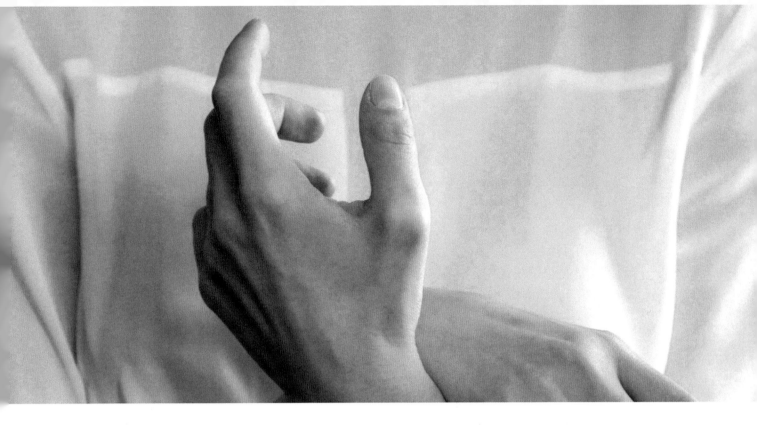

Instructions

To have the best results, all these tasks that I recommend in this guide are **to be done daily and consistently for 6 weeks**. Yes, I know that seems like alot, but DeQuervain's is a serious and complex injury that requires time to begin improving.

Performing some tasks will be straight forward, such as wearing a brace, others such as the exercises, I want you to do within your tolerance. The harder is not the better.

The exercises also have additional information on how many repetitions and times per day you should do them.

Finally, we will be going over activity modification. That is just a fancy way of saying I will teach you the general understanding of how to change the way you are performing your everyday tasks so they are safer for your hands and wrists (to further help decrease pain and prevent future injury). I won't be able to go into the specifics of your life, but by understanding these general "rules" you will understand how to safely perform YOUR EVERYDAY TASKS.

Week 1

The Equipment
You Need

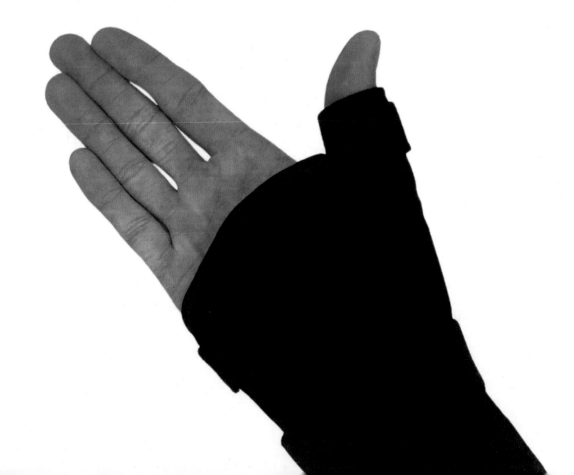

It doesn't matter who you are, where you come from. The ability to triumph begins with you. Always.

OPRAH WINFREY

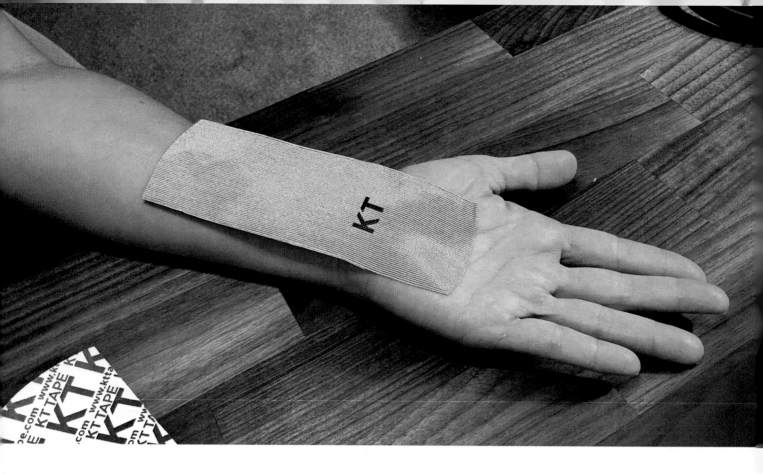

Week 1

The Equipment You Need

The goal of this week is to get you started and to get you used to being on a program.

I know starting this program feels overwhelming. It is alot, but it is for a very valuable reason: YOUR HEALTH! YOUR LIFE! YOU!

Remember that as you continue working!

You got this week! Woohoo!

Tasks To Do This Week

1. Wear a brace during the day and at night.

2. Kinesiotape

3. Wear an edema glove

1. Wrist Brace

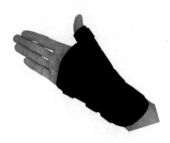

Wrist brace wear is one of the major players in preventing, decreasing and managing pain and discomfort in the hand and wrist because it forces REST- exactly what an overused, overworked and in pain body part needs. But, how hard is it to force our hands and wrists to rest? Next to impossible without the brace!

Often times those I work with will say that they have already "tried" wearing the brace and it hasn't done anything for them. What I usually find out is that they haven't worn it enough. And also keep it mind that it is a "part" of the solution-NOT THE WHOLE SOLUTION!

Here are recommendations for braces to make getting and starting to wear a brace easier. Luckily these braces come from Amazon so if you don't like how it feels on you, return it and contact me. We will find something that fits you.

1. Wrist Brace

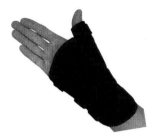

Suggested braces (find on Amazon):

For daytime wear (wear ideally all day):

a. Curecare New Updated Thumb Brace

For nighttime wear choose one of the following (wear while you are sleeping):

a. Rolyan D-ring Wrist and Thumb Spica Splint

b. Braceability Thumb and Wrist Spica Splint

c. Thumb Spica Splint & Wrist Brace

The above items are affiliates meaning if you purchase one of the splints, I will receive an affiliate commission at no extra cost to you. This, however, does not influence which braces I recommend to you.

Wear schedule:

The recommendation is to wear your brace while you are sleeping (because that allows for multiple hours of resting your hand and wrist) and during the day, ideally all day (for the first 4 weeks). After 4 weeks, if symptoms are decreased and controlled, you only have to wear the night splint. I know that sounds like alot and next to impossible, but try your best! Let me know if this becomes too challenging. I can help you find a way!

Tips:

1. Do not tighten the straps too tight (wear snug but not too tight). The tighter is not the better! You should be able to slide a finger into both ends of the brace.

2. Wear a thin sock underneath your splint to make it more comfortable to wear (cut a hole at the top for your fingers and a side hole for your thumb).

3. Wear a sock on top of your brace so the velcro straps don't get caught on anything! And same thing, cut a hole at the top and a hole on the side for the fingers!.

2. Kinesiotaping

Kinesiotape can be used to help with many different problems: pain, swelling, muscle tightness, nerve compression, lymphatic flow and muscle imbalance to name a few. When kinesiotape is stuck to the skin and we move the body part that is taped, it's stretch and recoil properties move the skin and the layers of tissue underneath. This can cause and/or influence mechanical and/or chemical processes in the hands and wrists (and any other body part). We then get a decrease in our symptoms.

Kinesiotape is great in that it can benefit in so many different ways but it is not invasive and gentle. Anyone can use it!

Here below is a way to "tape" yourself. Here is a link to the kinesiotape I recommend (it is also on the resources page). Using kinesiotape can be tricky at first so please contact me if you have any questions!

Wear schedule: Once you have taped yourself, wear for 24-36 hours (if it starts to loose alot of stickiness or it's uncomfortable remove before the 24-36 hours). Kinesiotape is water proof. If there is some unraveling in the corners than cut that part off and re-adhere the rest.   Wear underneath your brace at night. To remove, remove in the shower or bath and remove gently. Replace again after allow your skin to breathe for 20-30 minutes.

2. Kinesiotaping

- Start by cleaning with soap and water the area you will be taping. In this case the hand, wrist and forearm of the injured side/sides. Thoroughly dry.
- Cut one strip of kinesiotape that is the length of a little more than the length of your forearm. (As you continue to use kinesiotape, you will get to know the length of kinesiotape that you really need. For now it is better to go longer and have excess than the other way around.)
- Cut a slit about one inch down the middle of one end of the strip. It doesn't matter which end you cut. Refer to the picture.

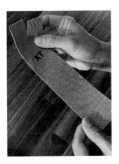

- Now cut all corners (both ends of the tape) so they are more rounded including the corners of the cut you made down the middel. Again, refer to the picture.

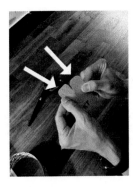
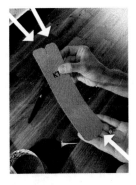

- Flip over the tape and tear across the tape at the end that has the slit. Tear across right below the slit.

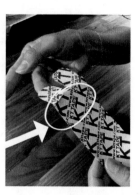

- With the tape still flipped over, now remove the smaller paper back (the end closer to the slit).

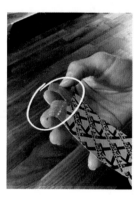

- Now flip the entire tape over and wrap the slits end around your thumb. Scratch the tape. This helps to stick the tape even better to you.

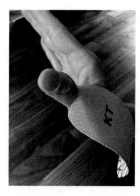 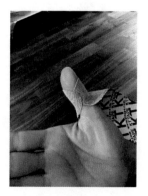

- Now place your hand on a supportive surface (table, etc.).

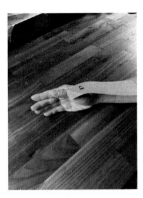

- Remove the rest of the paper backing on the tape. Make sure to keep the tape from sticking on itself.

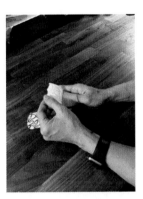

- While holding the end of the tape with the uninjured hand, raise the thumb of the injured side towards the ceiling.

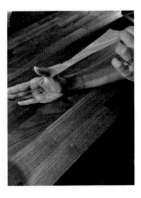

- Now while giving the tape a slight stretch, stick the other end of the tape in the direction of the elbow (as far as it will go with only a slight stretch to the tape-DO NOT STRETCH THE TAPE ALL THE WAY!). Remember to keep the thumb raised as you are placing the other end of the tape. DO NOT YET STICK DOWN THE ENTIRE LENGTH OF THE TAPE-JUST THE END!

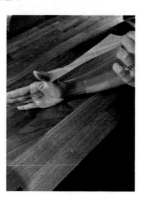

- These are pictures of how it would look with the end placed down. These are pictures from different angles. PLEASE NOTE THAT I HAVE YET TO STICK DOWN THE MIDDLE PART OF THE TAPE!

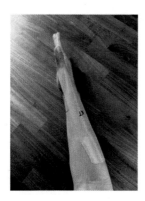 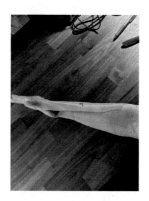 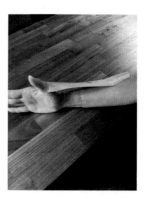

- Now gently bend your wrist sideways down as comfortably as you can go.

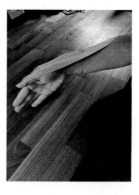

- Now rub along the ENTIRE LENGTH of the tape to tape it to your arm. Then scratch along tape to additionally make sure it is stuck to your arm.

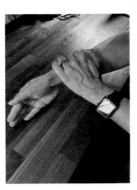

- Good job!! You did it! This is how it should look. These are pictures from different angles.

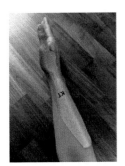 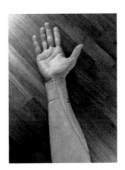 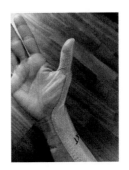 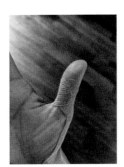

3. Edema Glove/ Edema Management

Edema is a fancy word for swelling or retaining fluid in the body/in a body part.

Typically when there is injury to a body part, in this case due to overuse or overworking the hand and wrist, the body will react with some swelling.

Swelling is not all bad. It is the body's way of beginning to heal an injured area. But more swelling than what is expected or swelling that is not being removed by the body can cause problems-stiffness with trying to move the hand and wrist and scar tissue/adhesions which all lead to pain.

So we want to manage and decrease swelling in the hand and wrist as much as possible! Here are two things you want to start doing:

3. Edema Glove/ Edema Management

1. Edema Glove:

An edema glove is a glove that gives light compression (it feels like a gentle hug to your hand!) to your hand and wrist. It is important in that it helps to discourage swelling from just "sitting" in your hands and wrists. My patients often tell me how good it feels. **Wear at night under your brace.**

Here is a recommended one for you (click on the name/link):

Rolyan Compression Glove

You can choose either the style that covers your fingers or ones that don't. It is entirely up to you.

The above links are affiliate links meaning if you click on the links and purchase one of the splints, I will receive an affiliate commission at no extra cost to you. This, however, does not influence which braces I recommend to you.

2. Edema massage: (this is optional)

Holding your affected hand up (ideally, place your elbow on a table with your hand up) and using lotion, use unaffected hand to give gentle pressure/massage to affected hand. Move in the direction of fingertip down towards elbow (NOT in the other direction-see picture A). Do for approx 5 minutes, 3 times per day. DO NOT DO if you have any heart condition or medical conditions involving your veins. Check with your doctor.first.

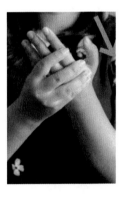

Picture A

Tips: Make sure that your glove is not too tight. To test this, make sure that when you are wearing it, your finger tips are not turning abnormal colors, your fingers are not going numb and that you can slide a finger under the glove easily.

REVIEW

01 Wear a brace daily! This is a significant part of your recovery because it forces the hands and wrists to rest. If you are having a hard time finding one you can wear, contact me!

02 Kinesiotaping is a handy and effective tool to have in the management of your pain.

03 Edema/swelling is a normal part of injury to the body. However, we don't want to allow it to sit there because that can cause pain and other problems!

Tasks Completed
For Week 1

	M	Tu	W	Th	F	Sa	Su
Wear my brace day and night.	○	○	○	○	○	○	○
Kinesiotape.	○	○	○	○	○	○	○
Edema massage	○	○	○	○	○	○	○
	○	○	○	○	○	○	○

	M	Tu	W	Th	F	Sa	Su
	○	○	○	○	○	○	○
	○	○	○	○	○	○	○
	○	○	○	○	○	○	○
	○	○	○	○	○	○	○
	○	○	○	○	○	○	○

	M	Tu	W	Th	F	Sa	Su
	○	○	○	○	○	○	○
	○	○	○	○	○	○	○
	○	○	○	○	○	○	○
	○	○	○	○	○	○	○
	○	○	○	○	○	○	○

Hi my friend!

I am so proud of you for just starting this week.
So whatever you completed or didn't complete, know that because you tried, you deserve the biggest hug of congratulations.
Thank you for putting your health first this week. Because your health should never be on the bottom.

With love,
Rose

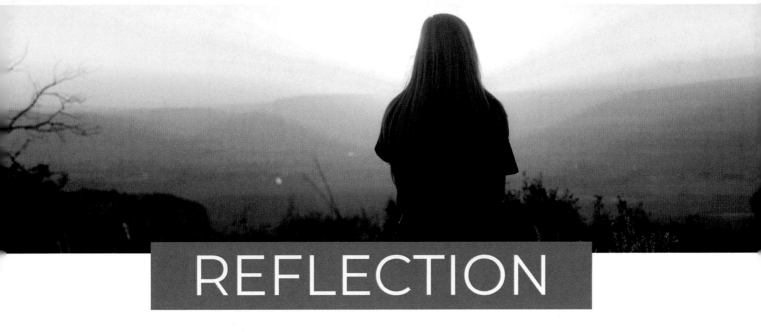

REFLECTION

Use this page to reflect on your week. Don't just focus on the highs and lows of decreasing your pain, but focus on life as well. If you'd like, share it with me and our community on our online group. I would love to hear about your thoughts!

_____
_____
_____
_____
_____
_____
_____
_____
_____
_____
_____
_____
_____
_____
_____
_____
_____
_____

Week 2

All About Soft

Tissue Work

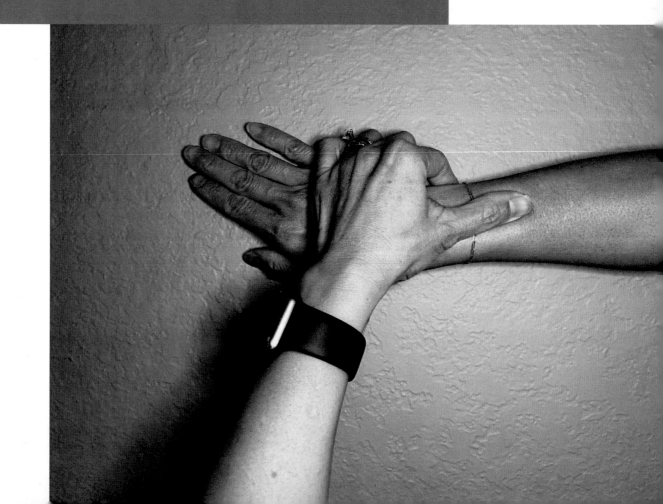

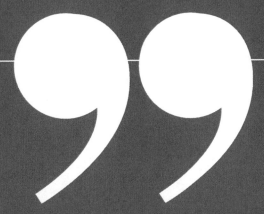

Never underestimate the power you have to take your life in a new direction.

GERMANY KENT

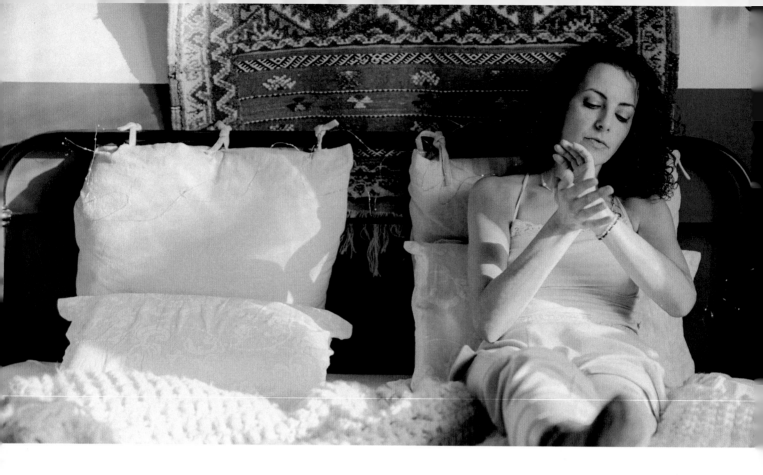

Week 2

All about Soft Tissue Work

The goal of this week is to progress you a little further now that you have begun to get used to doing a home program.

Something you keep in mind as you continue with this guide is that it is cummulative, meaning you will continue with all the prior week's/weeks' tasks as you start the new week. So for this week, remember to continue last week's tasks.

Don't start to get worried about how much you will be doing though! True, getting better takes dedication and time, but do the best you can! And I'm here for you!

Tasks To Do This Week

1. Wear a brace during the day and at night.

2. Kinesiotape.

3. Wear an edema glove.

4. Perform soft tissue work daily.

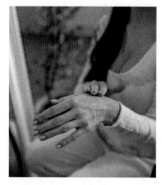

1. Soft Tissue Massage (STM)

Soft tissue massage is about reducing pain and tightness in muscles and fascia, improving circulation, decreased swelling and breaking down scar tissue/adhesions. More often STM is not really relaxing at all! But it is so important to have it be a part of your program.

Massage in a circular fashion each spot shown below (the circled areas) for about 3 minutes, 3 times a day. Use lotion to make it more comfortable. Try to give yourself as deep of a message as you can tolerate.

Pro tip: Make sure to cut your nails!

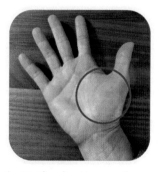

At the bottom of your hand

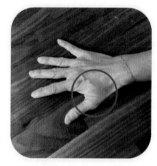

Space between your thumb and index finger

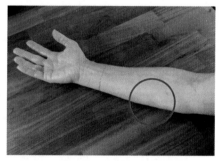

By your inner elbow

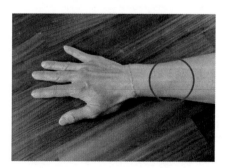

About this distance from your wrist

2. Instrument Assisted Soft Tissue Massage (IASTM)

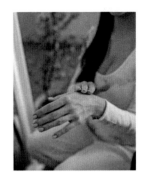

A step further of how we can perform the above soft tissue massage is to use an "instrument" (either the handle of a butter knife or a spoon) to help break down adhesions and soften the fascia (tissue that surrounds the insides of our body).

What you will do is massage all the spots shown above (and below) with the handle of a butter knife or a spoon (it is up to you to decide which is more effective and comfortable).

How to do it: Angle the insturment to the spot you will be working on. It should be at about a 45 degree angle to the area. Giving medium pressure, glide the instrument over the area, changing directions every minute. Do for 3 minutes, 3 times a day. Use lotion to make it more comfortable. Do as tolerated. If you have problems or questions please feel free to contact me!

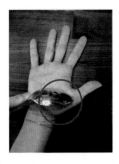

At the bottom of your hand

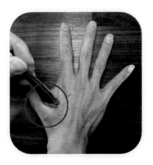

Space between your thumb and index finger

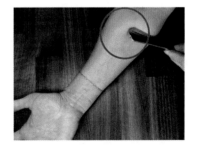

By your inner elbow

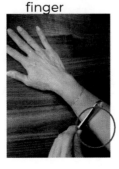

About this distance from your wrist

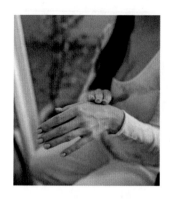

3. Pin and Stretch Technique

Pin and stretch technique is used to help lengthen tendons, restore glide of tendons and to help break up adhesions between the tendons and other tissue. All of this means healthy movement of the tendons involved in DeQuervain's which in turn means less pain!

During pin and stretch, you will be "pressing" on ("pinning") the muscle belly of the tendons that we are focused on as you move the corresponding body part. Then you will end with a little deep tissue gliding massage. This might be confusing at first so please feel free to contact me.

Work on each of these areas for about 3 minutes, 3 times per day. Use lotion.

A. Into wrist flex and ext:

-The movement: The movement the injured hand will be doing during this technique is as below: 1. Start with the hand of the injured side raised to the ceiling by bending at your wrist (picture A). 2. Alternate with bringing the hand of the injured side down by, again, bending at your wrist (picture B).   You will alternate between these two movements as your uninjured hand is "pinning" and performing the gliding massage.

-The "pinning" and gliding massage: Referring to picture C, these are the "x's" where you will be "pinning" (or pushing down on) with your uninjured thumb. You will push down on the first "x" as your injured hand is moving from position A->B. Then once your injured hand is in position B you will do a short massage "gliding" towards the next "x" in the direction as shown (picture D). Continue in this fashion until you reach your elbow (or the last "x") (picture D). You don't have to be exact with the "x" locations.   Basically you want to "pin" on those general spots.

-Do this for 3 minutes.

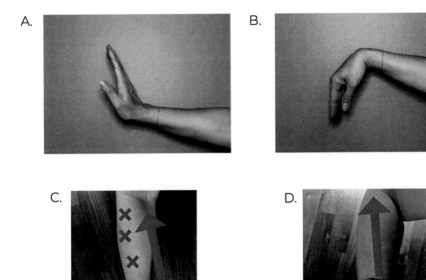

A. Into wrist radial and ulanr deviation:

-The movement: The movement the injured hand will be doing during this technique is as below: 1. Start with the hand of the injured side bent sideways towards the thumb side (picture A). 2. Alternate with the hand of the injured side bend towards the pinky side (picture B). You will alternate between these two movements as your uninjured hand is "pinning" and performing the gliding massage.

-The "pinning" and gliding massage: Referring to picture C, these are the "x's" where you will be "pinning" (or pushing down on) with your uninjured thumb. You will push down on the first "x" as your injured hand is moving from position A->B. Then once your injured hand is in position B you will do a short massage "gliding" (you will be putting medium pressure) towards the next "x" in the direction as shown (picture D). Continue in this fashion until you reach your elbow (or the last "x") (picture D). You don't have to be exact with the "x" locations. Basically you want to "pin" on those general spots.

-Do this for 3 minutes.

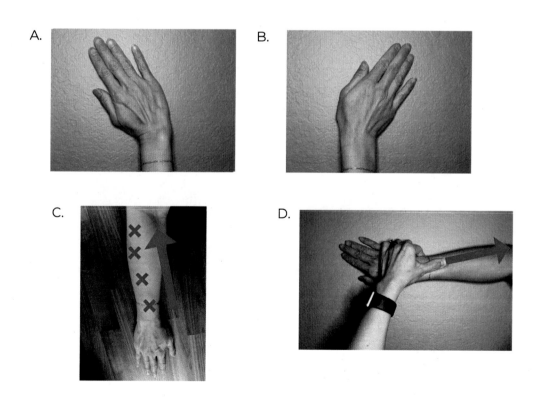

REVIEW

01 Performing soft tissue working is an important part of your therapeutic program. It not only helps to break down adhesions and tightness, but it encourages normal movement and speeds healing!

Tasks Completed For Week 2

	M	Tu	W	Th	F	Sa	Su
Wear my brace day and night.	○	○	○	○	○	○	○
Kinesiotape.	○	○	○	○	○	○	○
Edema massage	○	○	○	○	○	○	○
	○	○	○	○	○	○	○

	M	Tu	W	Th	F	Sa	Su
Soft tissue massage	○	○	○	○	○	○	○
Instrument assisted soft tissue massage	○	○	○	○	○	○	○
Pin and stretch	○	○	○	○	○	○	○
	○	○	○	○	○	○	○
	○	○	○	○	○	○	○

	M	Tu	W	Th	F	Sa	Su
	○	○	○	○	○	○	○
	○	○	○	○	○	○	○
	○	○	○	○	○	○	○
	○	○	○	○	○	○	○
	○	○	○	○	○	○	○

Hi friend,

I know that all the tasks are starting to add up and this guide is starting to ask alot of you. I know it's definitely starting to feel like alot of work. But please know that this isn't forever. There is an end in sight.

For right now, always congratulate yourself on the daily wins and the steps YOU ARE taking. Don't look at what you didn't get done, but rather see how far you have already come.

Looking at you with pride and love,
Rose

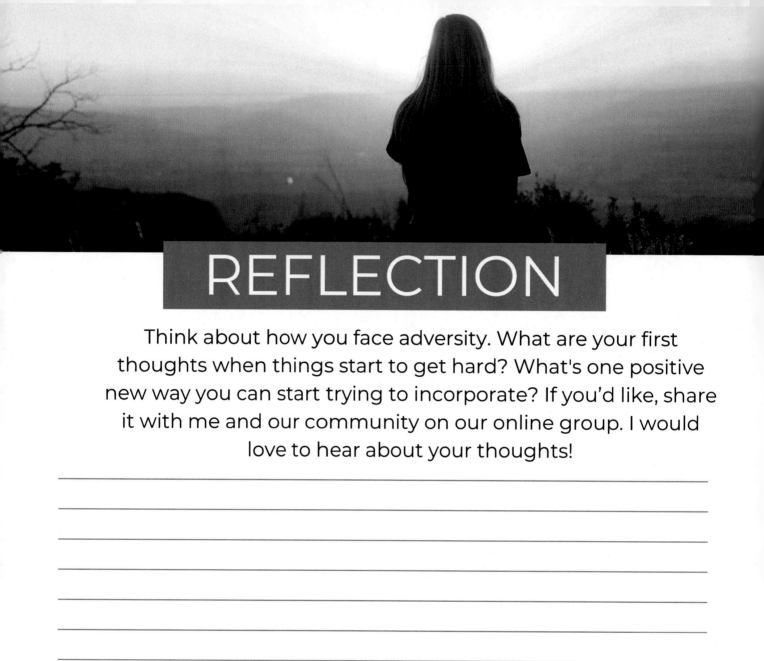

REFLECTION

Think about how you face adversity. What are your first thoughts when things start to get hard? What's one positive new way you can start trying to incorporate? If you'd like, share it with me and our community on our online group. I would love to hear about your thoughts!

_____
_____
_____
_____
_____
_____
_____
_____
_____
_____
_____
_____
_____
_____
_____
_____
_____

Week 3

Let's Get Moving

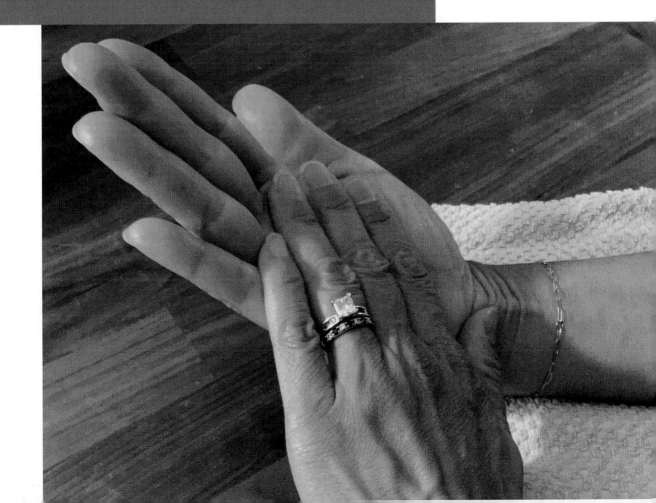

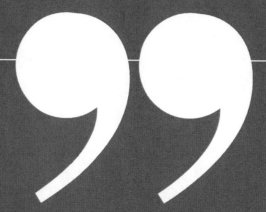

Optimism is the faith that leads
to achievement.

HELEN KELLER

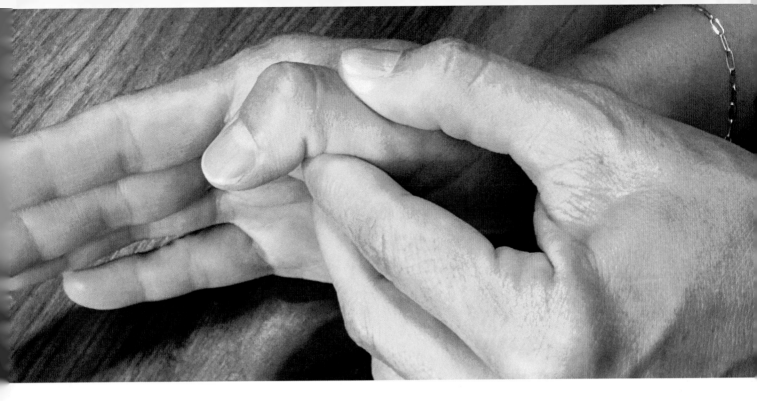

Week 3

Let's Get Moving (Range of Motion)

I know that the last thing you want to do when you are in pain is to move, especially in the direction that hurts! And yes, at this point in your recovery it is important to limit how often we are moving the hand and wrist into the painful direction, but WE DO STILL NEED TO MOVE IT IN THAT DIRECTION.

Range of motion, or exercises that actively move our body, not only helps to prevent stiffness and weakness, but also helps to encourage circulation of blood, oxygen and fluids in addition to preventing adhesions and scar tissue. What this all means is that it helps to heal our body and prevent further injury!

Tasks To Do This Week

1. Wear a brace during the day and at night.

2. Kinesiotape.

3. Wear an edema glove.

4. Perform soft tissue work daily.

5. Range of motion exercises.

Range of Motion

Instructions: As you are doing these exercises, challenge your pain level so you feel like you are progressing yourself, however DON'T OVERDO IT!! We don't want it to be very uncomfortable or very painful. THE HARDER IS NOT THE BETTER!

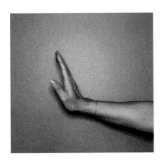

1. Active Range of Motion

Active Range Of Motion Exercises: Active range of motion means the body part is simply moved. Make sure to perform within your tolerance.

- **Tendon Glides**: Moving through each of the positions below is considered one round. Do a total of 3 rounds.

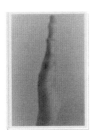 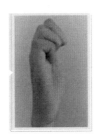 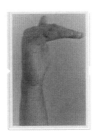 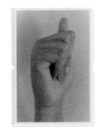 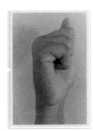

- **Thumb joint blocking IP joint (top segment of thumb)**: Thumb joint blocking MP joint (bottom joint of injured thumb): With the uninjured hand, hold below the bottom joint of the injured thumb (below the crease and not too tightly) as the picture shows (picture A). Now bend and straighten the bottom joint of the injured thumb (picture B). Return to starting position (picture A). Do 10 times, 3 times per day.

A.

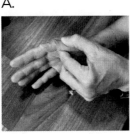

B.

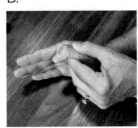

- **_Thumb joint blocking IP joint (top joint of injured thumb)_**: With uninjured hand, hold below the top joint of the injured thumb (below the crease and not too tightly) as the picture shows (picture A). Now bend and straighten the top joint of the injured thumb (picture B). Return to starting position (picture A). Do 10 times, 3 times per day.

A.

B.

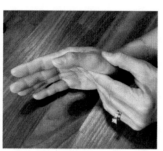
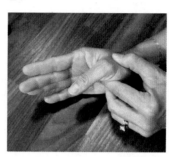

- **_Thumb slides_**: Start with your hand open (picture A). Slide your thumb down the face of your pinky finger (picture B and C) and then return back to open hand (picture A). Do 10 times, 3 times per day.

A.

B.

C.

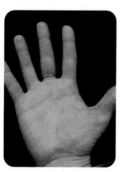
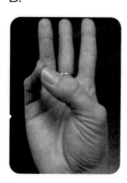
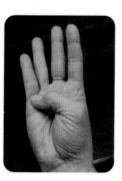

- **_Opening and closing the hand_**: Starting with your hand open (picture A), close the hand (picture B). Return to starting position (picture A). Do 10 times, 3 times per day.

A.

B.

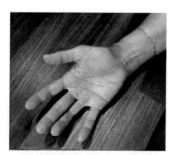
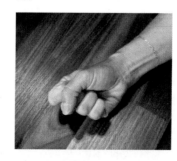

- **_Finger abduction/adduction_**: Start with fingers together (picture A). Spread fingers apart (picture B) and bring back together (picture A). Do 10 times, 3 times per day.

A.   B.

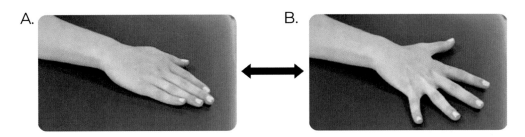

- **_Wrist circles_**: Do large wrist circles 10 times in one direction and 10 times in the other direction. Do three times per day

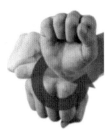

- **_Wrist side-to-side_**: Move hand side to side (like you are waving) 10 times. Do three times per day.

A.   B.

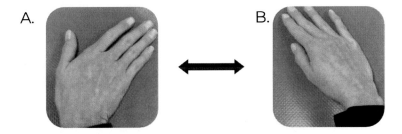

- **_Forearm supination and pronation_**: Start by having your arm by your side and bending your elbow to 90 degrees (as showin in both pictures). Then rotate your palm up (picture A) (while keeping your elbow by your side) and then rotate your palm down (while keeping your elbow by your side) (picture B). Do 10 times, 3 times per day.

A.   B.

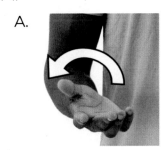 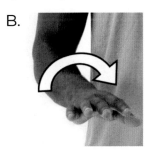

2. Passive Range of Motion

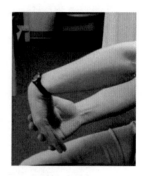

Passive Range Of Motion Exercises: Passive range of motion means the body part is stretched to the comfortable max it can go. Do gently and to your tolerance.

- *Prayer stretch/reverse prayer stretch*: Start by pushing the palms of your hands together until a stretch is felt (picture A). Hold 3 seconds. Then push backs of hands together until a stretch is felt (picture B). Hold 3 seconds. Hold each position 3 times. Do 3 times per day.

A. 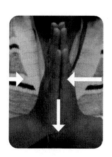   B.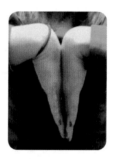

- *Forearm and wrist stretch*: Starting with stretching the arm of the injured side out in front of you. Use the hand of the uninjured side to gently push on the palm of the injured side towards your body. Hold for 5 seconds (picture A). Release. Then, again, stretching the arm of the injured side out in front of you, use you the hand of the uninjured side to give the hand of the injured side a gentle push on the back of the hand towards your body (picture B). Hold for 5 seconds. Alternate back and forth until you have done each position 3 times. Do 3 times per day.

A. 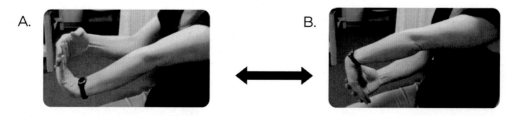 B.

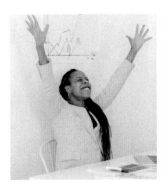

3. Range of Motion For The Upper Body

Our hands and wrists are an extension of our upper body so we need to make sure that our upper body is in good health too in order to keep our hands and wrists pain and injury free!

- **Neck stretches**: Rotate your head as the picture shows. Do 10 times in one direction and ten times in the other. Do 3 times per day.

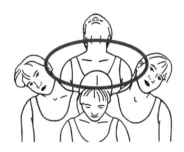

- **Back and neck stretch**: In a seated position, cross one leg over the other, twist your body over the crossed leg as if you are trying to look over your shoulder. Hold for 5 seconds. Rest and alternate legs and twist in the other direction. Hold for 5 seconds. Rest. Do 3 times in each direction. Do 3 times per day.

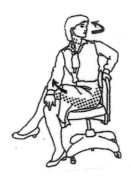

- **_Shoulder rolls_**: move shoulders in circular direction in one direction 10 times and in the other direction 10 times. Do 3 times per day.

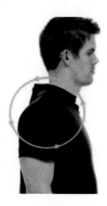

REVIEW

01 Range of motion is so important to start though it may cause discomfort. In fact, it helps with our recovery and preventing further pain!

Tasks Completed For Week 3

	M	Tu	W	Th	F	Sa	Su
Wear my brace day and night.	○	○	○	○	○	○	○
Kinesiotape.	○	○	○	○	○	○	○
Edema massage	○	○	○	○	○	○	○
	○	○	○	○	○	○	○
Soft tissue massage	○	○	○	○	○	○	○
Instrument assisted soft tissue massage	○	○	○	○	○	○	○
Pin and stretch	○	○	○	○	○	○	○
	○	○	○	○	○	○	○
	○	○	○	○	○	○	○
Active Range of Motion Exercises	○	○	○	○	○	○	○
Passive Range of Motion Exercises	○	○	○	○	○	○	○
Upper Body Range of Motion Exercises	○	○	○	○	○	○	○
	○	○	○	○	○	○	○
	○	○	○	○	○	○	○

I wish you could feel just how proud of you I am right now! I am bursting!!

It's only been three weeks, but it's felt like a long three weeks. I know. And I hope you are already starting to feel some relief, but if not keeping hanging in there and have faith. Faith in this program but mainly faith in yourself, that you will get yourself there. I have faith in you! As long as you keep working at and being the Superwoman that you are, you will get there!

With so much pride in you,
Rose

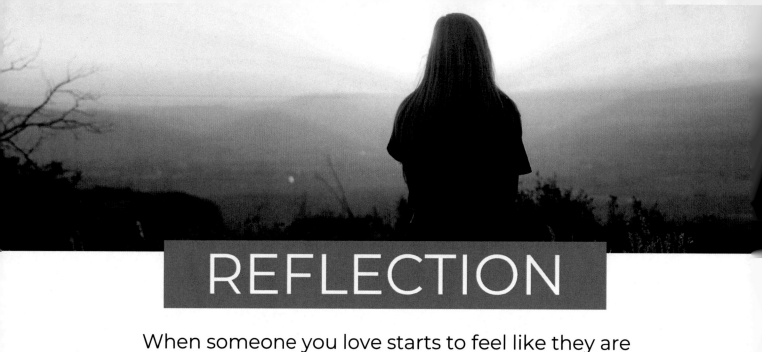

REFLECTION

When someone you love starts to feel like they are hitting a wall with their goals, what do you say? How do you keep them going?   Do you think those are words you should say lovingly to yourself? :) If you'd like, share it with me and our community on our online group. I would love to hear about your thoughts!

_____
_____
_____
_____
_____
_____
_____
_____
_____
_____
_____
_____
_____
_____
_____
_____

Week 4

Safe Performance Of Your Everyday Tasks

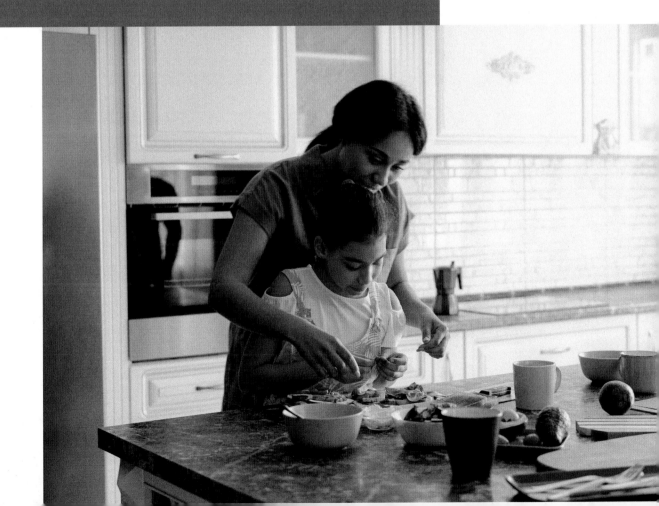

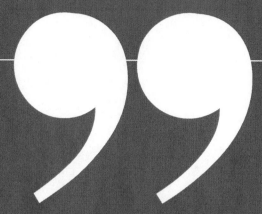

It doesn't matter how slow you go as long as you don't stop.

CONFUCIUS

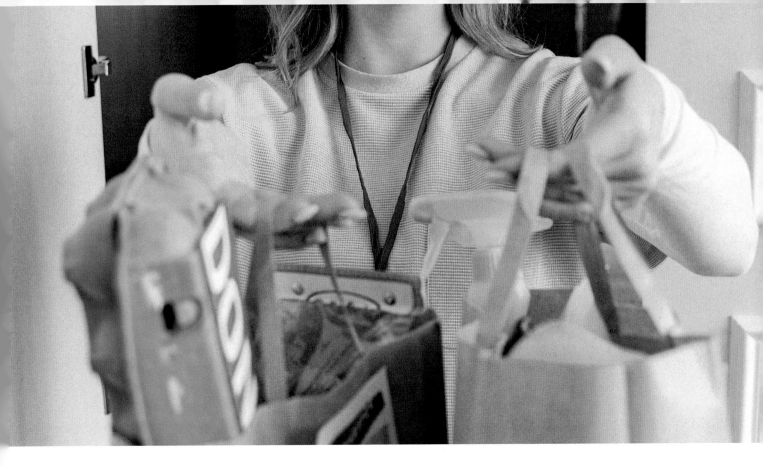

Week 4

Safe Performance of Your Everyday Tasks

I know it's been alot up to this point. I've given you ALOT of information in the last three weeks.

So for this week I won't be giving you additional exercises. We will just continue the ones we've been doing so far so we can get more comfortable with them. But make sure you are continuing with them!

This week, instead, will be about learning how to do our everyday tasks safer so we don't continue injuring our hands and wrists.

Tasks To Do This Week

1. Wear a brace during the day and at night.

2. Kinesiotape.

3. Wear an edema glove.

4. Perform soft tissue work daily.

5. Range of motion exercises.

Tasks To Do This Week

6. Perform everyday tasks safer to prevent injury and pain to the hands and wrists.

1. Let's Start With These Two Gems Of Advice

When I am asked "What are two things I can do to help with my thumb and wrist pain (DeQuervain's)?" this is what I say. Of course I know that when someone is asking me this they are expecting exercises, equipment, maybe even advice on what to be taking or eating.

But these two recommendations I have really are practical and powerful. They help with prevention, management and prevention of a reoccurrence.

Of course, these two things aren't the only things you should be doing, but they should definitely be included!

Actually, these two tips work with all overuse injuries!

• Take a break every 20-30 minutes

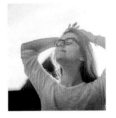

This is one of the best pieces of education I can give! It is the best thing to help decrease and prevent pain and injury.

I like to explain it like this: as we are using our hands and wrists everyday, we are causing microtrauma to it. As time continues (during our day) the trauma adds up. If we don't let too much time pass (a.k.a. we take a break) then not as much trauma has accumulated and the body is better able to heal and heal itself.

But, if we let too much time pass before we take a break, then the body isn't able to handle all that damage that has added up and then we end up with permanent injury and then pain. Always remember that we are not machines. Our bodies cannot handle doing activities for an extended period.

BUT TAKING A BREAK DOESN'T MEAN STOPPING WHAT YOU ARE DOING ALTOGETHER!

Taking a break, ideally, would mean lettting the body fully rest. But we're busy, so that's not always an option. So the other ways we can "rest" the body is by using equipment to help us perform the activity or performing the activity a different way (for example, use the other hand/wrist to do it or approach it with different mechanics/posture/alignement-more on this later).

Tips:

1. Remember it's not about stopping an activity or activities altogether. It's about NOT DOING AN ACTIVITY FOR A SUSTAINED OR LONG DURATION.
2. Set up ways to force yourself to take a break: set an alarm on your phone, drink alot of water so you'll have to go to the bathroom often...be creative!
3. When you take that break, do a quick stretch to your body, do a quick walk around the room...something to give your body a chance to breathe!

• Stretch your body open!

Majority of the activities that fill our life demands us to bend our neck down, collapse our chest inward, bring our arms in, bend at our wrist and grip/close our hand.

So we need to balance that out by opening into the opposite direction as below.

Spending too much time in one position can lead to muscle weakness AND muscle tightness, stress on joints and ligaments and compression to nerves. What this all equates to is PAIN!

The Movement:

Go back and forth between these two positions slowly.
Hold for 3 seconds, do 3 times, do it 3 times a day.

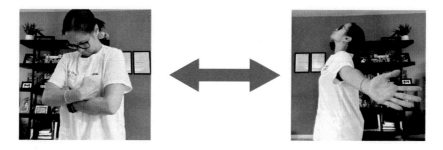

Position 1: Bend your head down, keep your arms by your side, bend your elbows, bend your wrists and close your hands.

Position 2: Bend your head back, stretch your arms towards your back (opening up your chest), bend your wrists back and open up your hand (and stretch out your fingers).

Tips:

A good way to remember to do your exercises is to do it at meal times. That way if you ate, you know you did your exercises. Or find a specific time of the day that works for you. The important thing is to do it the same time every day. This way it becomes a habit.

2. Let's Talk About Alignment

Why is alignment so important when it comes to DeQuervain's?

With any overuse injury, as the name implies, we are OVERUSING OUR BODY. Overusing our body can mean working it for an extended period, forcing it to exert too much effort or putting it in positions for also an extended period. How ever you are overusing your body, it all results in damage and pain.

Now what is alignment? In regards to our hands, wrists and forearms, we are talking about these parts being in a relatively straight line with each other and the rest of the arm and upper body. One of the reasons alignment is important is that it allows these smaller body parts (i.e. hands, wrists, thumbs) to be able to get assistance from larger body parts (arm, shoulder, trunk) for things such as strength.

And why is this important? It is actually VERY IMPORTANT! Alignment helps our body perform activities with less effort and with less stress. What this means is less damage to our body.

- Keeping your head, neck, shoulders and trunk aligned.

I know it's strange to be mentioning the head, neck, shoulders and trunk, but what I have always taught and continue to teach my clients is that the hand and wrist are not isolated. They are part of a larger chain that connects to the rest of the body. So the proper alignment of the head, neck, shoulders and trunk is important in keeping the hand and wrist functioning well (and forearm, elbow and upper arm actually).

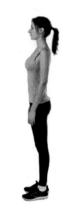

This is a good example of an ideal alignment of your head, neck, shoulders nd trunk- everything is stacked on top of each other.

Without taking a deep dive into details, making sure that you keep your head aligned with your neck aligned with your shoulders and aligned with your trunk (in a seated or standing position) helps your hands and wrists to be able to function, move through it's full range, to have the best mechanical advantage and to be assisted by the larger muscles of the upper arm and trunk/core.

Keep this in mind when doing such activities as nursing your child (I will talk about the ideal position later) and working at your work station (I will also talk about this more later). Keep this in mind while standing at the kitchen counter or working out or doing any activity.

So, overall, make sure you are watching your posture with whatever you are doing!

It's hard to list all activities that are a good example of when to incorporate this tip, but if you have a question for an activity specific to your life, contact me or post in our Facebook community.

- Keeping your shoulders, elbows, forearm, wrists and hands in a neutral position when holding items by your side.

When we carry things such as bags by our side it is best to carry it with our shoulders, elbows, forearms, wrist and hands in the neutral position (picture A). When we carry items by our side like in picture B below it puts alot of stress (that then leads to pain) on the hands all the way to the shoulders because it does not allow larger muscles to assist.

A.

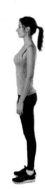

This is a good neutral position.

B.

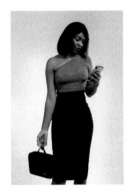

This is a NOT a good way to hold a bag because it is not in neutral position

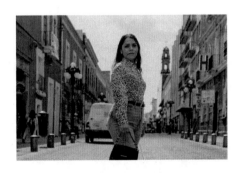

This shows a good neutral position while holding a bag.

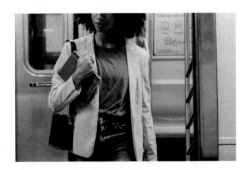

However, this IS THE IDEAL way to hold your purse or bag because the larger muscles of the arm and trunk help.

- ## Keeping your hands aligned with your forearms.

This is a power move for decreasing your hand and wrist pain.

The hand and wrist are some of the smallest body parts on your body so making sure that they are assisted and supported by the larger body parts is important. We are able to do that when we keep the hand and forearm aligned (the hand and forearm are keep in a straight line as much as possible) while doing activities as much as possible. Do keep in mind that I understand there are times when you can't keep the hand and forearm aligned. And that is ok. Just try to keep them aligned as much as possible throughout your day.

So what does this exactly mean?

Here are examples of how your hand and wrist should and should not be positioned while doing activities:

How your hand and forearm should be:	**How your hand and forearm should not be:**
Hand and wrist kept in a relatively straight line to each other	Hand and wrist not in a straight line relative to each other

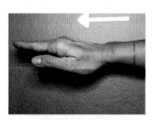 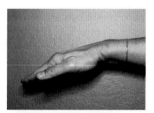 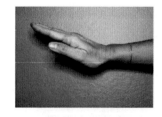

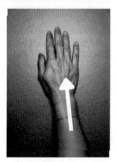 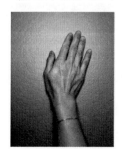 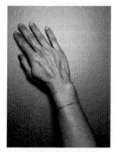

Activities that give you an idea of how you should and shouldn't position your hand and forearm relative to each other:

- ***Holding our child/children.***

More often than not, caregivers will hold their children where one or both of their hands are NOT in alignment with their forearms. Repeatedly doing this for weeks, months or even years will aggravate the tendons involved in DeQuervain's (amongst other structures) and lead to injury. I know it's hard to change this habit, however, try to be more aware and try to definitely change the position of your hand and wrist when your body begins to become fatigued and uncomfortable. DON'T JUST POWER THROUGH! We will talk more about safe child holding later on.

How you should:
Hand is in line with forearm

How you shouldn't:
Hand not in line with forearm

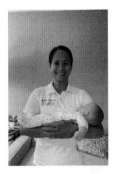 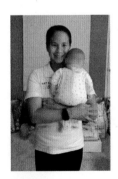 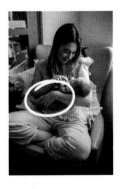 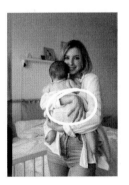

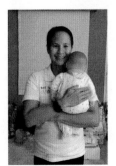

- **_Working at your computer workstation._**

Often times our workstations are not set up to support keeping our hands and wrists in alignment with our forearms (workstation set up will be discussed in more detail later). For example, our entire body should be supported so that we can easily keep the forearm in line with the hand while typing (we shouldn't have to work hard at keeping our hand and forearm aligned). AND while we are typing, we should limit how much we raise our hand up in order to type-even if we raise our hands up minimally. Finally, if you have been wondering, no, wrist rests are not helpful. Actually they can cause problems by putting pressure on the nerves that run through our wrists.

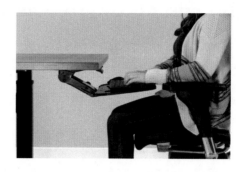

This is actually an example of an ideal set-up!
We will discuss more about what you need to set-up an ideal work station later.

- **_Using your cell phone._**

Without realizing it we are also setting up our hands and wrists for pain when we poorly use our cell phones. I very hardly see a person scrolling or texting in a way that is safe for their hands and wrists. The ideal position is to make sure your hand and forearm are in a straight line as best as possible. The extra benefit is that you are holding your cell phone more upright which is better for your neck! I will recommend additional tips on how to hold and use your cell phone to, again, protect your hands and wrists later on.

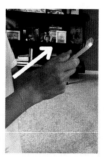

How you should hold a cell phone: *hand and forearm in a straight line*

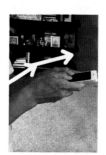

How you shouldn't hold your cell phone: bend at wrist (even if it's slight)

- # Keeping your thumb close to the other four fingers.

I like to call this the "Barbie" (or any doll really) hand. And eveyone knows what I mean by that! It means you keep your fingers close together. However, I am more specifically focused on the thumb. We often have a tendency to hold items with our thumb stretched out to give a more secure hold and more often than not it is unnecessary or avoidable.

The reason I am focused on this is if you remember back to the beginning of this guide, the tendons in DeQuervain's are irritated when we hold our thumb away from the rest of the four fingers either repeatedly or for an extended period.

So when you can, try to keep your thumb close to the rest of the fingers! Again, I know there will be moments when it is impossible and that is ok. For the rest of the times, do the best you can!

How you should hold your thumb:
Close to the rest of the four fingers

How you shouldn't hold your thumb:
Away from the rest of the four fingers

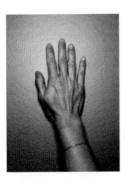

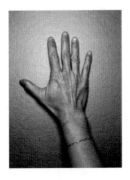

Activities that give you an idea of how you should and shouldn't position your thumb:

- ***Holding our child/children.***

Often times when we hold our children we will spread our thumb out to give an extra hold on them. Like I mentioned this is unncesary. We can still hold them securely with our thumb placed next to our index finger (Please only do this if you feel secure holding your child this way.). These are examples below:

| *How you should*:
keep your thumb close to the rest of your fingers | *How you shouldn't*:
thumb spread from rest of fingers |

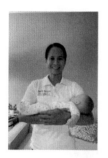 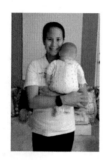   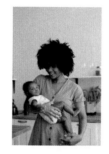 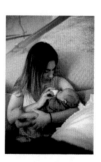

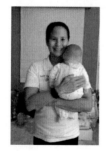

- ***Holding our cell phones***

Going back to how we hold our cell phones, we can also improve how our thumb is positioned. Now I know you are wondering, how we can do that without dropping our phones!! And yes, you're right, you can't without dropping it. And that's why I love cell phone rings or cell phone holders. Any of them work, doesn't matter the style or brand. It's just using them. Because then it allows you to hold your phone without overworking the hand and thumb!

How you should: keep your thumb close to the rest of your fingers

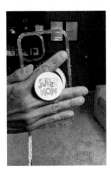

How you shouldn't: thumb spread from rest of fingers

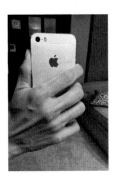

- **Texting or scrolling on our phone**

I know it sounds lame to do it this way, but truly this is another highly recommended tip to keep your thumb and wrist safe and injury free. Often times we scroll/text on our phones with the same hand that is holding the phone. This puts alot of stress on the tendons involved in DeQuervain's.

I highly recommend holding the phone with one hand, while scrolling and texting with the other as follows:

How you should: using one hand hold the phone while the other scrolls/texts

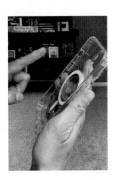

How you shouldn't: using one hand to scroll/text on your phone

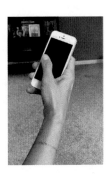

Again, I will come back to how we can improve using our cell phones because it is such a common and repeated activity in our day. So stay tuned!

3. Tips for Everyday Activities

Now I want to give you general tips for everyday activities and examples of them so you can further have a general understanding of how to modify YOUR everyday activities to protect your hand and wrist from injury.

I know some of these tips and examples will still seem confusing. It really is hard to take an example and apply it to your life and specific activities. That's my job! So please feel free to contact me!

- ## Always use larger muscles as much as possible.

Which muscles are your larger ones when it comes to your hands, wrists, forearms, arms and shoulders? As you move from your hands towards your shoulders, your muscles become larger (and, hence, stronger). Therefore when you can, you want to try and avoid using the muscles within your hands (these can be more easily damaged in addition to the other structures in your hands).

What would that look like?

That means trying to not hold things with your hands. Rather you want to use your forearm, arms and shoulders. Here are a few good examples:

- ***Carrying a bag or purse***

Hopefully you are already familiar with NOT carrying your bag/purse with your hand for a long period (it's ok if it's for a few seconds or minutes). Carrying it on your forearm or on your shoulder or, ideally, on your back is better.

How you should: holding bag/purse on your forearm, shoulder or back

How you shouldn't: holding bag/purse with your hand

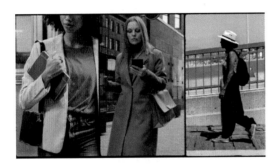

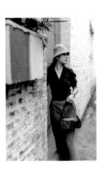

- ***Carrying items***

It is ideal to carry items (especially if they are heavy) underneath (therefore using larger muscles) rather than carrying items with your hands. By making sure to do it this way then you will not overwork your hands and wrists.

How you should: carrying item from underneath

How you shouldn't: carrying items with your hands

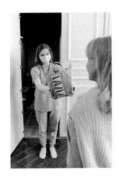

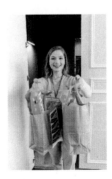

- ***Pushing heavy items***

When possible push items with your arm and not your hand. For instance, push open a door with your arms, close a door also with your arms.

How you should: pushing with your arm or body

How you shouldn't: pushing with your hands

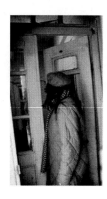

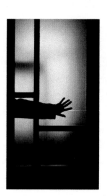

- Gripping with less intensity when possible.

When possible (and safe) you want to try and grip whatever you are working with/holding with the least amount of effort as possible. Generally, we hold items alot tighter than we need to and, hence, that fatigues and stresses the hand and wrist and can lead to injury.   For example:

- Loosen your grip on your cell phone.
- Loosen your grip on your pen/pencil/mouse/cooking or eating utensil/etc.
- Steering wheel (when safe).
- See if you can loosen the grip on your child when holding them (it is up to you to decide when and if this is safe).

- ## Use better ergonomically designed versions of equipment and tools you use every day.

Now what do I mean by that?! That means that there may be a better designed version of a tool you use regularly that makes it easier for the hand and wrist to use. Now not everything has an ergonomic version, but for items that you use frequently it is worth a shot to see if there is one available. Also look at my resource page in the back of this guide for links!

- Use a wider pen like Dr. Grip (this can be found on Amazon). These take less effort to hold while using them.
- Use pens that are not too slippery or too thin. These take much more effort to hold while using them.
- If you cannot find a pen that you like, then you can take a pen that you do like and make it wider by adding coban wrap. This also helps make the pen less slippery. This can also be found on Amazon.
- As mentioned, have a cell phone ring or holder (like a pop socket) attached to your phone so you don't have to grip as hard.
- Certain cell phone covers make holding your cell phone easier because it adds texture to your phone that makes gripping it much, much easier. That means less effort for your hands.
- There are so many modified versions of everyday tools that we use! Take a look on Google or Amazon. Also take a look at my resources page in the back of this guide. Contact me also if you have questions!

- Change your position if you find yourself performing a task in an awkward (a.k.a. painful) way.

I cannot tell you how many times I've had clients tell me that it hurts when I do this this way (Yes, it's that cliche joke!). And no, my answer is not "Than don't do that." Well, it kind of is. LOL. What I typically tell my client is "Can you do it differently?" Majority of the time the answer is "yes".

I think that we get into the habit of doing something a certain way AND we are simply in a hurry to get it done, we ignore how uncomfortable our hand and wrist (and other parts of our body) are. Try repositioning yourself. And often!

4. Special Topics

Here are a few topics that I think need extra time and attention paid to. However, I know that there are a million, billion different activities out there that I am not able to touch on in this guide. Please contact me about any specific activities that you might have questions on!

Topics we will be talking about are:
- Holding your child
- Setting-up for breastfeeding/nursing
- Computer workstation set-up
- Cell phone use

• Holding your child

This an important topic for anyone with children in their life. Holding a child, especially for the long periods that he/she wants us to hold them, can be stressful and then, eventually, damaging to our body.

So it is important that I teach the safest way to hold your children that decreases the risk of injury to your hands and wrists. I will reference the three common holds.

For the following activities, I will show you the common hold and how I would recommend improving it. For these recommendations, it is your responsibility to decide for yourself if you feel safe holding your child as recommended for your hand and wrist health.

1.Cradle holding

This is a hold we do often in a child's first year of life (and sometimes beyond). It can very easily put stress on our hands and wrists because of the need to hold the child extra securely or because we need to position the child in a certain way (as in breastfeeding). The recommendations to improve safety to your hands and wrists are to always remember to position your thumb close to the rest of your fingers and to try to keep the hand and forearm aligned. Additionally, when you can, hold your child with both arms (then neither hand/arm has to bear the child's weight entirely). Finally, when you are cradle holding while feeding/nursing your child, I highly recommend using a nursing pillow or at the very least a pillow to support your child's body so the stress of holding your child's weight is not only on your hands and wrist. I will talk about recommendations for decreasing risk of hand and wrist pain with breastfeeding/feeding later on.

Typical hold	**Recommended improvement**

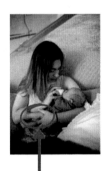 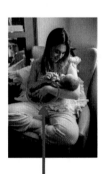

Thumb not close to rest of fingers

Wrist and forearm not aligned

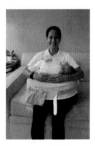

Hold hand and wrist in alignment. Thumb close to rest of fingers. Using pillow to support baby's weight.

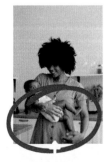

Not holding child with both arms

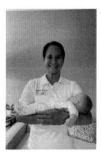

Hold hand and wrist in alignment. Thumb close to rest of fingers. Using both arms to support baby's weight.

2. Over The Shoulder holding

This is another hold we do often for the first few years of a child's life (and also beyond). It can also very easily put stress on our hands and wrists because of the need to hold the child extra securely and/or because of a growing child (getting heavier and longer).

The recommendations for this are the same: try to remember to keep your thumb close to the rest of your fingers and try to keep the hand and forearm aligned. With this hold, however, we have a tendency to hold the child's bottom with our forearm AND hand/thumb. This puts a TON OF STRESS to the hand and thumb. To avoid injury we need to make sure we have the child's bottom on our forearms and our hands are kept free. I always tell my clients that if you can wriggle your hands freely while holding your child (while the child is kept safe) then you're doing it right!

Typical hold	*Recommended improvement*
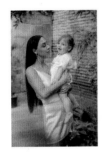 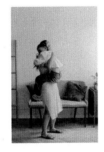	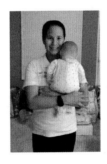 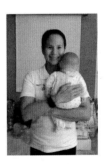
Wrist and forearm not aligned, thumb not close to other fingers, weight of child on hand and forearm	Wrist and forearm aligned, thumb close to other fingers, weight of child on forearm only

3. *Hip holding*

This a hold that I do not recommend. If you absolutely have to do it, then try to do it for a short period. It is a hold that forces one side to entirely hold the weight of the baby by itself (and remember, the hand and wrist have small muscles to begin with, so this is really not an ideal hold).   Additionally, this hold forces the spine out of alignment which then affects the neck and back (and really the ENTIRE body) AND it forces your shoulder to sit in an unnatural forward position. So though it is a seemingly easy and convenient way to hold your child, it really can lead to a variety of problems.

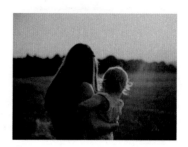

• Breastfeeding/feeding set-up

As caregivers we are taught so much about the proper way to breastfeed/feed our child. *But*, we are hardly ever taught how to breastfeed/feed our child so that we don't incur an injury to OUR hands, wrists, forearms, arms and shoulders. I believe it's a topic that needs to be taught more to caregivers because those injuries happen more often than caregivers and medical providers realize. And without this information, caregivers are getting these avoidable injuries!

So here are recommendations to make sure YOUR hands and wrists (and arms and shoulders too!) are staying as painfree as possible while breastfeeding/feeding your child.

1.Make sure that your entire body is supported

Again, we are often taught how to position the baby for breastfeeding/feeding so that the child is in the perfect position to latch or take the bottle. However, we are not taught the ideal position for us caregivers to protect our own body. And this is important because if your hands and wrists (and arms and shoulders and neck and back) are in pain, this sometimes challenging activity is made that much more difficult. We need to set you up to be as successful as possible and that includes taking care of you!

Now I know these recommendations I am about to give you might not always be do-able in certain situations. What I will say is to do the best you can and incorporate what you can because even those small changes help! When you are in a more ideal situation, for instance home, than make sure to do all the recommendations.

The following are recommendations. Try your best with them and contact me if you have any questions. However, you must keep in mind that you must **do what is best for your baby and you.**

1. Make sure to sit upright (no slouching). Have a pillow/pillows to support your back. You should feel like the pillows will securely hold you upright. YOU SHOULD NOT HAVE TO WORK TO HOLD YOURSELF UPRIGHT. If you have the right pillows (or other similar support) than you should be able to rest while the pillows do all the work holding you in the right posture.

2. Everything from the hips down to the feet should also feel supported. So you can either have your feet planted on the floor (which means you will have to sit forward in your chair (or whatever you are sitting on) or you can sit cross-legged. The important thing is your thighs need to be at hip height. Again, YOU SHOULD NOT HAVE TO WORK TO KEEP YOUR THIGHS HIP HEIGHT. IF YOU ARE SITTING PROPERLY AND SET UP PROPERLY THAN YOU WILL FEEL SUPPORTED FROM YOUR HIPS DOWN.

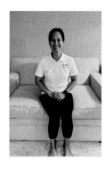 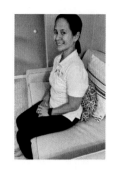 ***Proper positioning of the body for breastfeeding/feeding***: sitting upright (not slouching), thighs at about hip level, everything from hips down are supported and pillows behind your back

2. Make sure that you are using a truly supportive nursing pillow (or other supportive object)

A proper nursing pillow helps to make sure that you, your body and especially your hands and wrists do not have to work so hard to bring baby to the proper height and position for nursing/feeding. So a nursing pillow is not just for the baby, it's for YOU TOO! I know that there are situations where it is impossible to get a nursing pillow, so I recommend at least using some supportive object (for example, any pillow) to help support and hold your baby. That is better than not using anything!

If you do decide to use a nursing pillow, it is very important to be picky about what you choose. The type of nursing pillow you choose truly makes a difference. You want one that is sturdy (but not hard so that it is still comfortable for your baby) and maintains it's shape. That means it is not too soft that when you put your baby on it it just sags or deforms. YOU WANT IT TO HOLD YOUR BABY TO YOU OR TO YOUR CHEST SO YOU DON'T HAVE TO. The right nursing pillow will hold your baby at the right position and height for you so that all you have to do is have your hands nearby "just in case". I recommend the My Brest Friend (listed in resource page at the end of this guide) because it not only is sturdy (but still comfortable for baby), but it also has features like being able to strap it to you so that the nursing pillow stays securely where you need it to be throughout the feeding. This is very important because that means your hands and wrists (and arms and shoulder and body) don't have to work hard in keeping the pillow in place.

Here is an example of how a good nursing pillow should look:

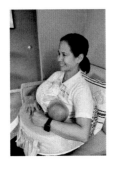 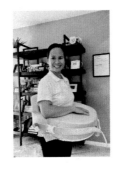 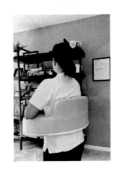 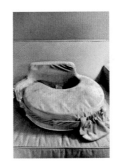

3. Make sure that you are watching the alignment and posture of your neck, shoulders, hands and wrists.

Often times when we are breastfeeding or nursing our baby we have a tendency to look down at them or our phones, cave in our shoulders and, finally, hold them close to us with our hands and wrists in poor alignment. This all contributes to injury and pain in our body including our hands and wrists.

Here are things we want to be aware of to change when we are breastfeeding/feeding our children:

1. It's okay to look at our baby while we feed them, but we want to make sure to do it only for a short period and then return to a good posture including looking straight ahead (which brings our neck back into a good neutral position). If we are looking at our phones, we want to make sure to hold our phones up to eye level instead of bring our heads down to where we are holding our phones. This is actually good advice for looking at our phones at all times.

2. We want to make sure that when we are seated while feeding our children, we are resting our entire back into the supportive pillows (meaning resting with good posture). You shouldn't have to hold your posture upright. You should be able to easily rest in an upright posture because you have set up your spot to be supportive of your body.

3. We want to make sure our hands and wrist are not in poor alignment while we are breastfeeding/feeding our children. Often times, as our child is feeding, we will unknowingly have a hold on our child that is not the best position for our hands and wrists. Or we will hold on our children so they do not roll off the nursing pillow with more exertion than is necessary to keep them safe, but this leads to discomfort and pain to our hands and wrists.

4. Try and loosen your grip as much as it is safe to. We often will overly hold an object or our child-more than is necessary. This will quickly fatigue your hand and wrist and lead to injury.

• Computer workstation set-up

This is an important topic to review as the majority of us are using a computer in some way, whether for work or personal use. Often times, too, we are working at our computers for an extended period (even though we should be taking breaks every 15-20-30 minutes!). It is important than to make sure you have your work station set up as best as possible.

Here are some important things to keep in mind:

1.Set up your workstation to support your entire body (including down to your feet).
I tell my clients that a general rule of thumb to know if your workstation is set up correctly is if you feel like your body is completely (or almost completely) supported by your workstation and workstation equipment. Your workstation and workstation equipment should be able to hold you upright and in a good posture. The only exertion should be by your fingers moving while typing. If you feel like you and your body has to exert effort to keep yourself in a good posture then something needs to be adjusted. Refer to the following picture and explanations to get a good idea of how to set up your workstation:

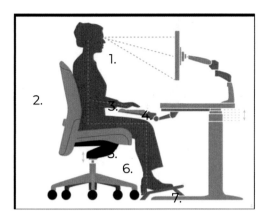

1. Eyes should be level with the top of your monitor. Make sure your head is in line with your shoulders.
2. Adjust chair back so that it is supportive and holding you upright (not tilted back/forward).
3. Forearms should be slightly below parallel to the floor. Ideally, your chair would have armrests to support your elbow/forearm, but if you don't have it that is ok.
4. Ideally, your keyboard is on a keyboard tray that is tilted down towards the desk (look closely at the picture). This helps to keep the forearm and hand aligned. Very important.
5. Your thighs should be about parallel to the floor.
6. There needs to be space between the back of your knees and the chair.
7. Your feet need to be supported-either on the floor or on a

You might have to experiment with different configurations, maybe even different styles of chairs, desks, footrests and monitors. You might even need to stack books underneath your monitor to get the right height. Be creative with trying to find a setup that works for you! And, of course, I am here so feel free to contact me if you need some recommendations!

Also, because many of us work from home and don't have access to a keyboard tray, here is an example of a set up without one.

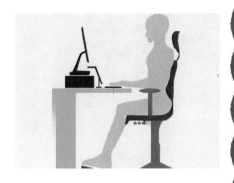

So following the same suggestions as the above workstation, the only thing you will change is raising up your seat so your wrists hover above your desk (your wrist should not touch the desk or anything!). Remember to keep your hand aligned with your forearm. In raising up your chair you might now need a footrest.

2. Use equipment that helps to keep your hand, wrist and forearm aligned and in a neutral position.

It's important to use equipment that helps keep the hand, wrist and forearm aligned because that means we are helping the hand, wrist and forearm to be in a less strained position (and less strained means less injury). The main equipment that I will discuss are:

1. The keyboard
2. The mouse

- *The keyboard*

A traditional keyboard forces the hands to be out of alignment with the forearm resulting in stress to the hand and wrists.

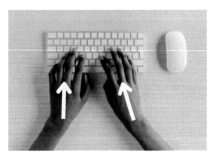

With use of a traditional keyboard the hands and forearms are not in a straight line (not aligned). This can lead to strain on the hands and wrists.

The keyboard that I recommend are split keyboards. Split keyboards allow the left and right side hand, wrist and forearm to each be placed in a way that keeps good alignment.

Samples of split keyboards:

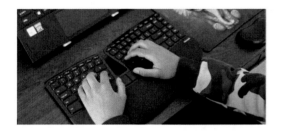 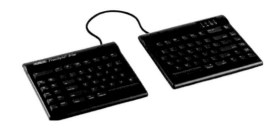

There is even one like this:

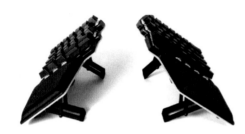

This is called a tented keyboard and they keep the hands, wrists and forearms in a more neutral position which means less strain.

- *The mouse*

The traditional mouse puts the hand, wrist and forearm in a strained position for multiple reasons. First it positions the hand, wrist and forearm in what is called pronation (that is the palm is down). This position strains the hands, wrists, and forearms because it stretches tendons, nerves, ligaments, etc.

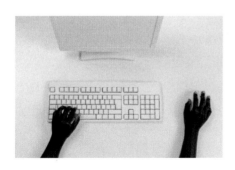

Hand, wrist and forearm position with a traditional computer mouse.

What we want is a mouse that places our hands, wrists and forearms in a neutral position.

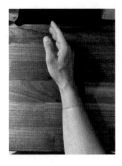

This is neutral position. This is the ideal position for mouse use.

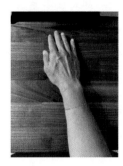

This is pronation. This is not ideal, however, this is the position with use of a traditional mouse.

So the mouse that I would recommend is something like this which is called a vertical mouse. This places the hands, wrists and forearms in the neutral position while using the mouse.

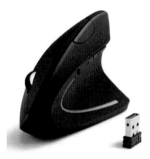

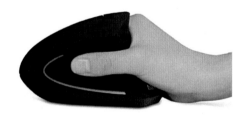

- Cell phone use

Now this is an important topic to review since for the majority of us this is an important part of our lives, hence, it is very important that I educate you on how to use it safely as to avoid hand and wrist injuries. Here are my recommendations on how to modify using your cell phone to protect your hands and wrists:

1. Use a cell phone cover

This is important to help you grip your phone better (that is if you pick one that decreases the slippery-ness of the phone). With a cover you will have an easier hold on your phone which means less need to overly grip your phone. This in turn helps to decrease the effort that your hand has to exert to hold the phone.

2. Use your cell phone with both hands
We already discussed this earlier, but I want to mention it again because it is so important!!

I highly recommend holding the phone with one hand, while scrolling and texting with the other as follows:

How you shouldn't: using one hand to scroll/text on your phone

How you should: using one hand hold the phone while the other scrolls/texts

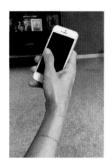
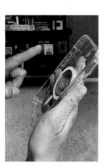

3. Use something to hold your cell phone better like a ring or something similar to a popsocket.
For the same reason as the cell phone cover, this helps your hand to not have to exert so much effort to hold the phone. In fact with these tools your hand really doesn't have to grip at all! Here are some examples:

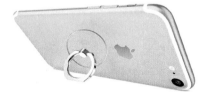
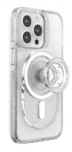
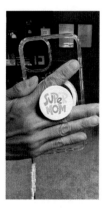

4. Watch the alignment of your hands and forearms while you use/look at your phone

Often times, we hold our phones in a way that is not ergonomically the best:

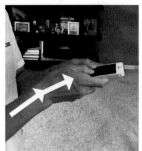

This is not good for your hands and wrists or your neck and back!

This is how you want to hold your phone:

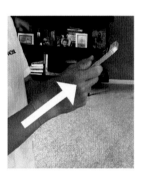

This is ideal. Additionally, try to hold it at eye level!

REVIEW

01   Take breaks every 20-30 minutes.

02   Make sure to stretch open your body often throughout the day.

03   Watch the alignment of your body while doing tasks.

04   Remember to perform tasks with your thumb close to the rest of your other fingers.

05   When doing your everyday things, try to use larger muscles as much as possible.

06   Try to grip items with less intensity if possible.

REVIEW

07 Find better ergonomically designed versions of equipment you use on a regular basis.

08 Change your position if you find yourself performing a task awkwardly.

09 Make sure you are holding your child in a way that does not put extra stress on your hands and wrists.

10 Be aware of how you are setting yourself up when breastfeeding/feeding your child.

11 Be aware of how you are setting up your computer workstation and what equipment you use.

12 Be aware of how you are using your cell phone.

Tasks Completed For Week 4

	M	Tu	W	Th	F	Sa	Su
Wear my brace day and night.	○	○	○	○	○	○	○
Kinesiotape.	○	○	○	○	○	○	○
Edema glove and massage	○	○	○	○	○	○	○
	○	○	○	○	○	○	○

	M	Tu	W	Th	F	Sa	Su
Soft tissue massage	○	○	○	○	○	○	○
Instrument assisted soft tissue massage	○	○	○	○	○	○	○
Pin and stretch	○	○	○	○	○	○	○
	○	○	○	○	○	○	○
	○	○	○	○	○	○	○

	M	Tu	W	Th	F	Sa	Su
Active Range of Motion Exercises	○	○	○	○	○	○	○
Passive Range of Motion Exercises	○	○	○	○	○	○	○
Upper Body Range of Motion Exercises	○	○	○	○	○	○	○
Become more aware and improve how I am performing my everyday tasks	○	○	○	○	○	○	○
	○	○	○	○	○	○	○

Hi friend!

I know this whole process of decreasing your pain is not an easy one! But you are doing it! And it's not about how fast you are doing it or being perfect at it. It's just about trying. Taking those steps. No matter how wobbly.

I continue to be amazed by your perseverance! It takes a strong woman to continue forward.

I am here cheering you on. I hope you can feel it!

Warmly,
Rose

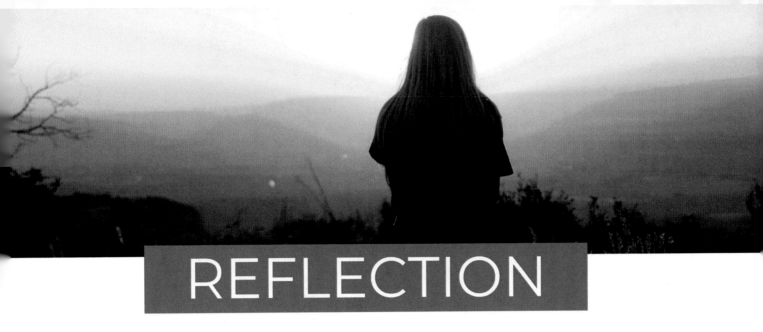

REFLECTION

How did this week feel? It was ALOT about keeping your body MOVING AND STRONG. But how do YOU feel? Do you feel like you are moving forward and do you feel strong (and I don't mean just physically) too? If you like, share it with me!. I would love to hear about your thoughts!

_____
_____
_____
_____
_____
_____
_____
_____
_____
_____
_____
_____
_____
_____
_____
_____

Week 5

Strengthen Your Foundation

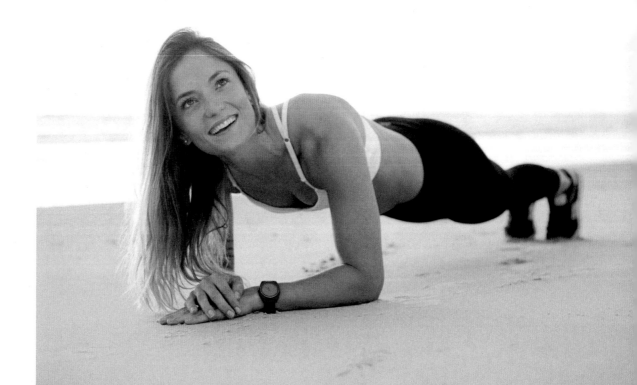

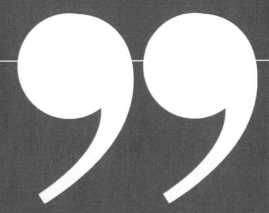

It always seems impossible until
it is done.

NELSON MANDELA

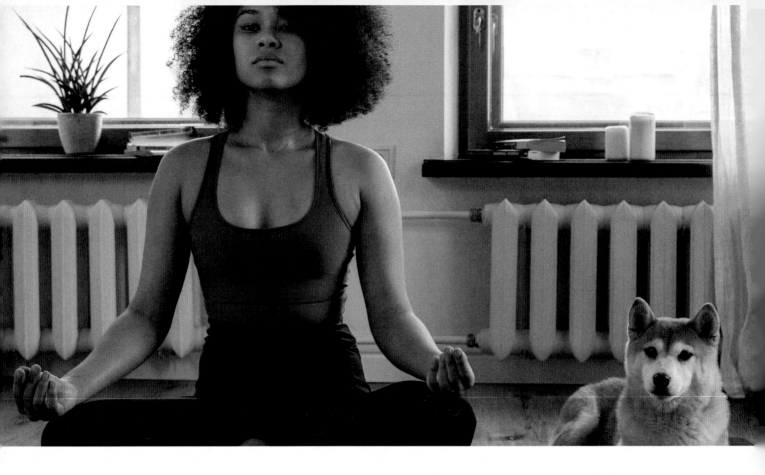

Week 5

Strengthen Your Foundation

Our hands and wrists are not isolated. They are connected to a larger chain that includes our shoulder girdle (which consists of our shoulder blade and our collar bone) and our trunk (which is our chest, our abdominals and our back).

The importance of that connection is that the health and function of the shoulder girdle and trunk affect how our shoulder, arm, forearm, wrist and hand function. It is, therefore, important to make sure that we are also working on the shoulder girdle and trunk in order to keep the hands and wrists healthy.

Tasks To Do This Week

1. Wear a brace during the day and at night.

2. Kinesiotape.

3. Wear an edema glove.

4. Perform soft tissue work daily.

5. Range of motion exercises.

Tasks To Do This Week

6. Perform everyday tasks safer to prevent injury and pain to the hands and wrists.

7. Strengthen the shoulder girdle and the trunk.

1. Let's Look At The Shoulder Girdle

The shoulder girdle. What is that?!

The shoulder girdle consists of the shoulder blade and the collarbone and is how the hand, wrist, forearm, arm and shoulder connect to the trunk and the rest of the body. They are all part of a long chain. The shoulder girdle, then, is influential to the function, range of motion and strength of the hands and wrists. It is, therefore, important to work on strengthening and mobility of the shoulder girdle.

Shoulder girdle exercises

- Shoulder circles: move shoulders in circular direction in one direction 10 times and in the other direction 10 times. Do 3 times per day.

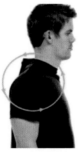

- Shoulder shrugs: bring shoulders up to ears 10 times. Do 3 times per day.

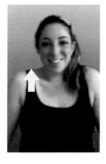

- Shoulder depression: push shoulders down to ground 10 times. Do 3 times per day.

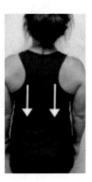

- Shoulder retraction: move shoulders(or arms) behind you 10 times. Do 3 times per day.

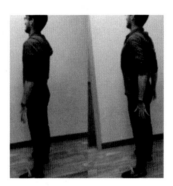

2. Now Let's Look At The Trunk

As mentioned the trunk includes the chest, abdominal and back muscles. These are the strongest muscles of your upper body. They also influence the function, range of motion and strength of the hands and wrists because they are the stable foundation from where the hands and wrists (and arms and shoulders) work from. These muscles hold the upper body still when the hands and wrists (and arms and shoulders) move. The hands and wrists will not be able to function well if the trunk could not hold itself still with strength and move through it's full range of motion.

Trunk exercises

- *Stretches*

1. In a seated position, cross one arm in front of your body towards the opposite shoulder. Hold for 5 seconds. Switch to the other arm, crossing over the body towards the other shoulder. Hold for 3 seconds. Do each direction 3 times, 3 times per day.

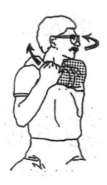

2. In a seated position, interlace your fingers behind you. As your fingers are interlaced, raise your hands up behind you (until you feel a stretch) while sitting tall. Hold for 3 seconds. Do 3 times, 3 times per day.

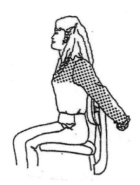

3. In a seated position, interlace your fingers in front of you. Raise your interlaced fingers to shoulder height. Push your hands out in front of you (like you are pushing someone who is in front of you). Hold for 3 seconds. Do 3 times, 3 times per day.

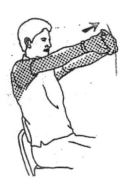

- *Strengthening*

  1. Upper Trapezius: Laying on your stomach on a supportive surface (place a rolled up towel under your foreheard to allow yourself to breathe), start with your arms by your side next to your thighs. Raise and lower your arms. Do 10 times, 3 sets, 1 time per day. You may do this holding a light weight or a small can/water bottle.

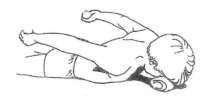

2. Middle Trapezius: Laying on your stomach on a supportive surface (place a rolled up towel under your foreheard to allow yourself to breathe), start with your arms out to your side (palms down) in line with your shoulders (like you are making a "T" with your body and arms). Raise and lower your arms (you don't need to raise it high). Do 10 times, 3 sets, 1 time per day. You may do this holding a light weight or a small can/water bottle.

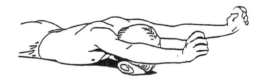

3. . Lower Trapezius: Laying on your stomach on a supportive surface (place a rolled up towel under your foreheard to allow yourself to breathe), start with your arms out in front of you (like you are Superman). Raise your arms up (you don't need to raise them high) and lower. Do 10 times, 3 sets, 1 time per day. You may do this holding a light weight or a small can/water bottle.

4. Scapular Depression: Sitting on a supportive surface with your feet flat on the ground (I know it doesn't show that in the picture, but make sure your feet are on the ground), place your hands (do with your hands gently fisted instead of open handed like the picture) on either side of you on the supportive surface. Push your hands down onto the supportive surface (like you are trying to push yourself up). Do 10 times, 3 sets, 1 time per day.

5. Serratus Anterior: Laying on your back on a supportive surface, raise your hands towards the ceiling (you will not be moving your hands up very much). Do 10 times, 3 sets, 1 time per day. You may do this holding a light weight or a small can/water bottle.

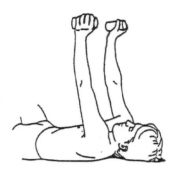

6. Scaption: Start in standing with arms by your side. Raise your arms towards the ceiling with thumbs up and elbows straight while making a "Y" with your arms. Do not shrug your shoulders. Return to the starting position. Do 10 times, 3 sets, 1 time per day. You may do this holding a light weight or a small can/water bottle.

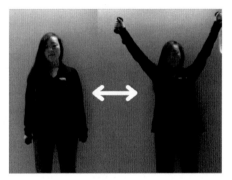

7. Sidelying External Rotation: Start in side-lying position, lying on side of uninjured arm, elbow bent to 90 degrees, place a towel under injured arm (see picture). Rotate injured arm so hand moves up towards the ceiling while keeping upper arm (of injured side) against towel and body (as shown in picture). Return to starting position. Do 10 times, 3 sets, 1 time per day. You may do this holding a light weight or a small can/water bottle.

8. Sidelying Internal Rotation: Start in side-lying position, lying on the side of the injured arm. DO NOT LIE ON THE INJURED ARM, rather have it close in front of you (see picture). Also bend elbow to 90 degrees. Rotate injured arm so hand moves up towards your body. Refer to picture. Return to starting position. Do 10 times, 3 sets, 1 time per day. You may do this holding a light weight or a small can/water bottle.

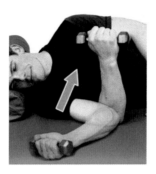

9. Abdominal Strengthening: Keeping your abdominals strong is also very important. The abdominals are a part of the trunk which again is the foundation that your hands and wrists work from. If you have any questions on which exercises to start with, you can contact me!

When it comes to choosing which exercises to perform for abdominal strengthening, finding a beginners program on the internet or on YouTube is a great place to start. Three exercises that I would recommend to start with are the following (as long as you feel like you can tolerate it):

- Plank pronated: While lying face down, lift your body up on your elbows and toes (picture A). Try and maintain a straight spine. Do not allow your hips or pelvis to drop. If you need to, you can modify this exercise by doing it on your knees (picture B). Actually you can modify it any which way that makes you feel challenged. Hold for 20 seconds, do 3 times, 1 time per day.

A

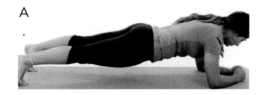

B

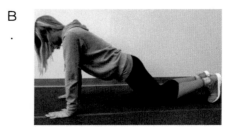

- Sidelying plank: While lying on your side, lift your body up on your elbow and feet (picture A). Try and maintain a straight spine. If you need to, you can modify this exercise by doing it on your knees (picture B). Hold for 20 seconds, do 3 times on each side, 1 time per day.

A.
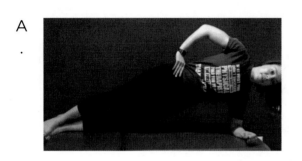

B.
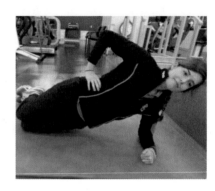

11. Yoga: Yoga is such a great way to work on overall strength, especially upper body strength. And it is great for any level because yoga can easily be modified. Go gently to start and stay within your tolerance. You can easily find yoga videos on the internet/youtube.

REVIEW

01 The health of the shoulder girdle and trunk is important in helping the hand and wrist to function well! We need to focus on these areas too!

Tasks Completed For Week 5

	M	Tu	W	Th	F	Sa	Su
Wear my brace day and night	○	○	○	○	○	○	○
Kinesiotape	○	○	○	○	○	○	○
Edema glove and massage	○	○	○	○	○	○	○
	○	○	○	○	○	○	○
Soft tissue massage	○	○	○	○	○	○	○
Instrument assisted soft tissue massage	○	○	○	○	○	○	○
Pin and stretch	○	○	○	○	○	○	○
	○	○	○	○	○	○	○
	○	○	○	○	○	○	○
Active Range of Motion Exercises	○	○	○	○	○	○	○
Passive Range of Motion Exercises	○	○	○	○	○	○	○
Upper Body Range of Motion Exercises	○	○	○	○	○	○	○
Become more aware and improve how I am performing my everyday tasks	○	○	○	○	○	○	○
	○	○	○	○	○	○	○

Tasks Completed
For Week 5

M Tu W Th F Sa Su

Perform exercises for the
shoulder girdle
Perform exercises for the
trunk

○ ○ ○ ○ ○ ○ ○
○ ○ ○ ○ ○ ○ ○
○ ○ ○ ○ ○ ○ ○
○ ○ ○ ○ ○ ○ ○

○ ○ ○ ○ ○ ○ ○
○ ○ ○ ○ ○ ○ ○
○ ○ ○ ○ ○ ○ ○
○ ○ ○ ○ ○ ○ ○
○ ○ ○ ○ ○ ○ ○

○ ○ ○ ○ ○ ○ ○
○ ○ ○ ○ ○ ○ ○
○ ○ ○ ○ ○ ○ ○
○ ○ ○ ○ ○ ○ ○
○ ○ ○ ○ ○ ○ ○

To my brave friend,

I simply just want to applaud you today.
Applaud all that you are doing. And
not just with improving your pain.

But with all that you are stepping up
and doing in your life. It's not easy, but
you're not backing down.

Bravo, bravo!

Warmly,
Rose

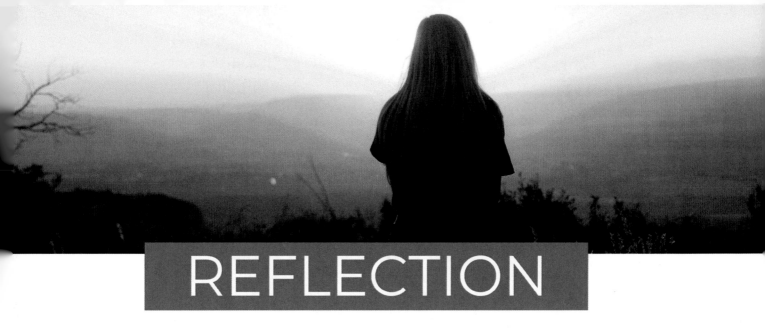

REFLECTION

Are you giving yourself moments to reflect on how far you've come? Or are you like me and don't give yourself enough credit? Write down all that you accomplished this week. And not just with this program, but with EVERYTHING! If you like, share it with me. I would love to hear about your thoughts!

_____
_____
_____
_____
_____
_____
_____
_____
_____
_____
_____
_____
_____
_____
_____
_____

Week 6

Strengthening

The Arms

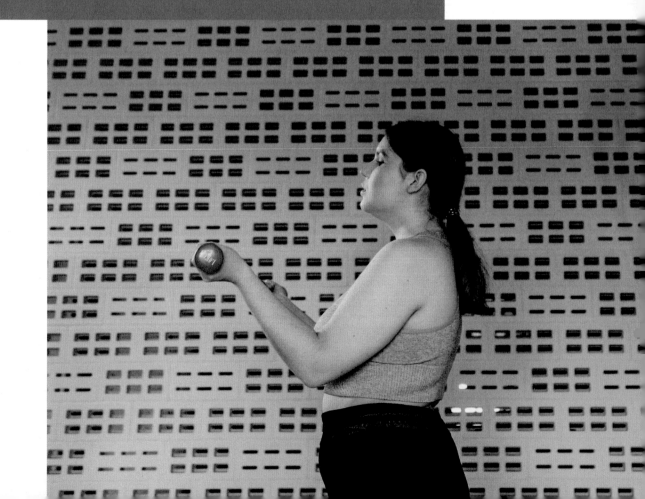

You're off to great places, today is your day.
Your mountain is waiting, so get on your way.

DR. SEUSS

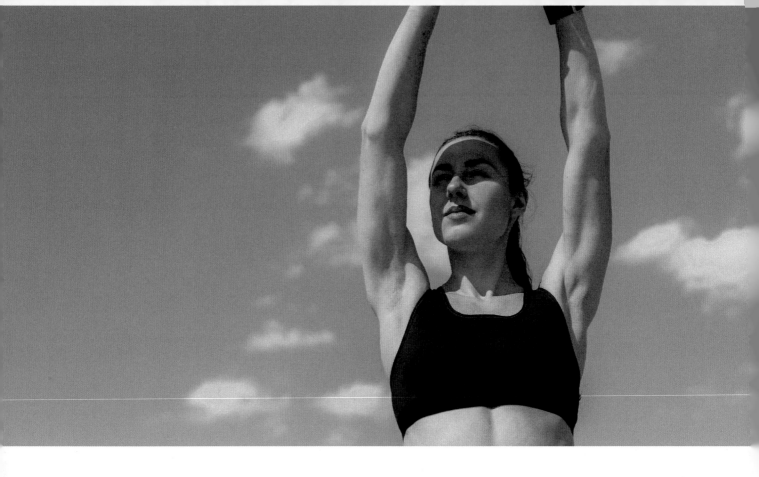

Week 6

Strengthening The Arms

Again, our hands and wrists are not isolated. They are part of a larger chain.

We've talked about the shoulder girdle and the trunk.

Now how about everything between those and the hands and wrists? How about the forearm, arm and shoulder?

These parts also are where the hands and wrists get function, strength and range of motion from. It is, therefore, important to work on the health of these areas.

Tasks To Do This Week

1. Wear a brace during the day and at night.

2. Kinesiotape.

3. Wear an edema glove.

4. Perform soft tissue work daily.

5. Range of motion exercises.

Tasks To Do This Week

6. Perform everyday tasks safer to prevent injury and pain to hands and wrists.

7. Strengthen the shoulder girdle and the trunk.

8. Strengthen the forearm, arm and shoulder.

Strengthening The Forearm, Arm and Shoulder

The parts of the arm between the shoulder girdle and trunk and the hand and wrist are important to strengthen as they are, too, a foundation of strength, range of motion and function for the hands and wrists. They literally help the hands and wrists to move in the direction you want them to in order to interact with the world.

Arm exercises

- Shoulder press: Start with arms as pictured (picture A). Then press/push your hands towards the ceiling as pictured (picture B). Return to starting position (picture A). You can either use light weights or a small can/water bottle. Do 10 times, 3 sets, 1 time per day.

A. 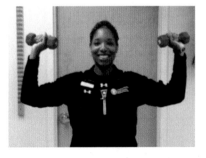   B.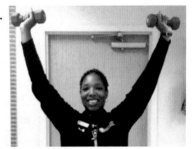

- Bicep curls: Start with your arms by your side as pictured (picture A). Then bend at your elbows to bring the weight towards your shoulders. (picture B). Return to the starting position (picture A) by slowly lowering your hands towards the ground. You can either use light weights or a small can/ water bottle. Do 10 times, 3 sets, 1 time per day.

A. 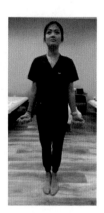 B.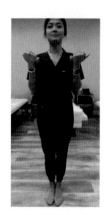

- Tricep extensions: Start with your arms as pictured (picture A)-the arm that is exercising will be bent at the elbow and supported by the other hand. Then extend the arm that is exercising at the elbow, bringing the hand towards the ceiling (picture B). Return to starting position (picture A). You can start with a light weight/small can/small water bottle if you feel safe doing so. Do 10 times, 3 sets, 1 time per day.

A. 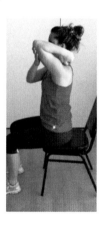 B.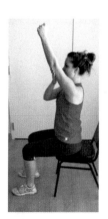

- Forearm pronation/supination: Rest your forearm on your knee or a table. Next, while holding the end of a small weight/small can/small waterbottle, slowly lower the weight towards the outside of your leg (picture A) and then rotate your forearm towards the inside of your leg (picture B). Go back and forth 10 times. Do 2 sets, 1 time per day.

A. 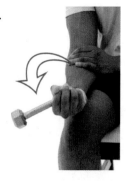 B.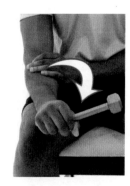

REVIEW

01 Keeping the forearm, arm and shoulder strong is also important for the hand and wrist to function well AND to avoid injury!

Tasks Completed
For Week 6

	M	Tu	W	Th	F	Sa	Su
Wear my brace day and night	◯	◯	◯	◯	◯	◯	◯
Kinesiotape	◯	◯	◯	◯	◯	◯	◯
Edema glove and massage	◯	◯	◯	◯	◯	◯	◯
	◯	◯	◯	◯	◯	◯	◯
Soft tissue massage	◯	◯	◯	◯	◯	◯	◯
Instrument assisted soft tissue massage	◯	◯	◯	◯	◯	◯	◯
Pin and stretch	◯	◯	◯	◯	◯	◯	◯
	◯	◯	◯	◯	◯	◯	◯
	◯	◯	◯	◯	◯	◯	◯
Active Range of Motion Exercises	◯	◯	◯	◯	◯	◯	◯
Passive Range of Motion Exercises	◯	◯	◯	◯	◯	◯	◯
Upper Body Range of Motion Exercises	◯	◯	◯	◯	◯	◯	◯
Become more aware and improve how I am performing my everyday tasks	◯	◯	◯	◯	◯	◯	◯
	◯	◯	◯	◯	◯	◯	◯

Tasks Completed
For Week 6

	M	Tu	W	Th	F	Sa	Su
Perform exercises for the shoulder girdle	○	○	○	○	○	○	○
Perform exercises for the trunk	○	○	○	○	○	○	○
Perform exercises for the forearm,	○	○	○	○	○	○	○
arm and shoulder	○	○	○	○	○	○	○

	M	Tu	W	Th	F	Sa	Su
	○	○	○	○	○	○	○
	○	○	○	○	○	○	○
	○	○	○	○	○	○	○
	○	○	○	○	○	○	○
	○	○	○	○	○	○	○

	M	Tu	W	Th	F	Sa	Su
	○	○	○	○	○	○	○
	○	○	○	○	○	○	○
	○	○	○	○	○	○	○
	○	○	○	○	○	○	○
	○	○	○	○	○	○	○

Hi my friend,

I know you are so exhausted. I know
you have done so much. And you
continue to do so much! Not just with
this program but for everyone around
you.

Take a rest, take a breath too, but don't
stop now. You are so close!

Rooting for you at the top of my lungs!

Warmly,
Rose

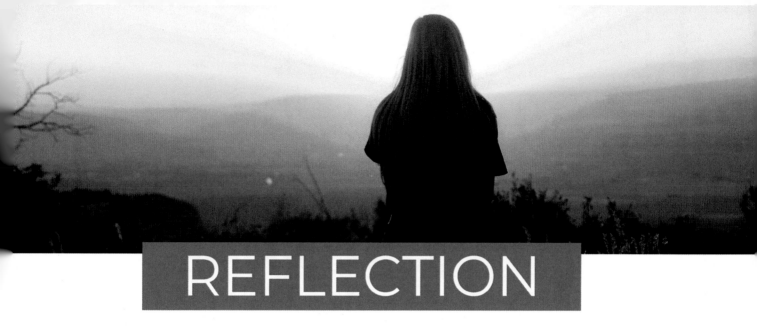

REFLECTION

Take a little self-assessment. How are you doing? How do you feel? What are the thoughts going through your mind right now? If you like, share it with me. I would love to hear about your thoughts!

_____
_____
_____
_____
_____
_____
_____
_____
_____
_____
_____
_____
_____
_____
_____
_____

Week 7

Strengthening The Wrists (Part 1)

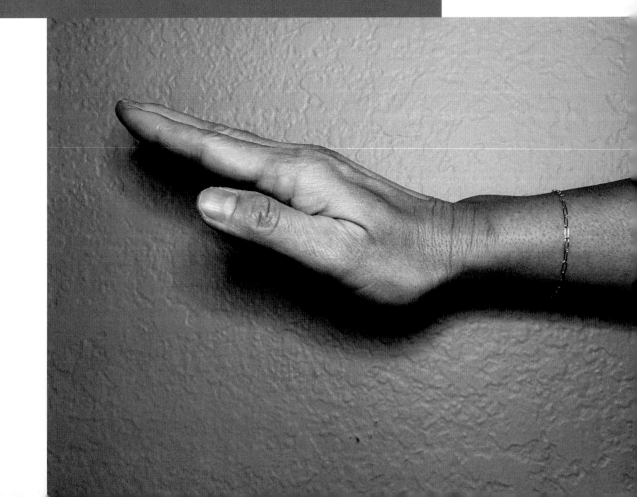

Believe you can and you're
halfway there.

THEODORE ROOSEVELT

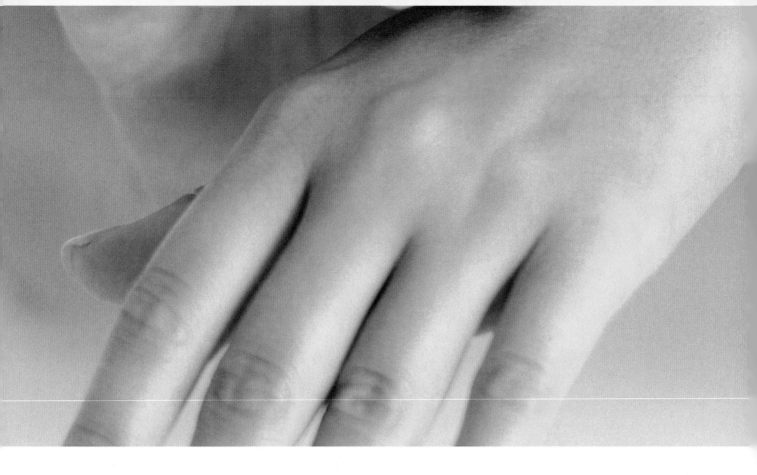

Week 7

Strengthening The Wrists (Part 1)

I get questioned often by my clients about why we don't strengthen at the wrists (and hands) right off the bat? Seems like that would be the logical first move right?

I actually tell my clients that if a therapist instructs you to strengthen the injured area right off the bat to run for the hills!

The injured body part should be slowly returned to strengthening.

So it's time. First let's start with the wrists!

P.S. A BIG CHANGE TO YOUR PROGRAM: WEAR YOUR BRACE JUST AT NIGHT!

Tasks To Do This Week

1. START WEARING YOUR BRACE JUST AT NIGHT.

2. Kinesiotape.

3. Wear an edema glove.

4. Perform soft tissue work daily.

5. Range of motion exercises.

Tasks To Do This Week

6. Perform everyday tasks safer to prevent injury and pain to the hands and wrists.

7. Strengthen the shoulder girdle and the trunk.

8. Strengthen the forearm, arm and shoulder.

9. Strengthen the wrist.

Strengthening The Wrists

Why are we only now strengthening the wrists?!

For two reasons: 1. The wrists (and the hands) are injured in the first place because they were overly stressed. Hence, the focus SHOULD NOT be on strengthening them initially (and stressing them more!). This would lead to further injury. 2. I like to explain the wrists (and the hands) as being at the end of a chain that depends on each other. Those at the end of the chain (the hands and wrists) can only function as well as those further up the chain (the arm, shoulder, shoulder girdle, trunk). Hence, it is important to strengthen at the trunk, shoulder girdle, shoulder, arm and forearm first before we even look at strengthening the hands and wrists.

Hopefully that all makes sense, but if you still have questions, contact me!

Wrist exercises

How we plan on strengthening the wrist will be different than what you are used to. The reason is is that these are less strenuous strengthening exercises for the hands and wrists and, hence, good starter exercises.

- Isometric wrist flexion: Start with arm and hand of injured side as pictured-wrist bent, palm raised towards ceiling (picture A). This is now hand A. Using the hand of the uninjured side (hand B), push down on the palm of hand A while hand A resists (hand A is trying to hold it's position). Hold for 3 seconds, do 3 times, do 1 time per day.

A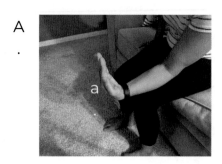

B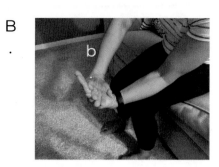

- Isometric wrist extension: Start with arm and hand of injured side as pictured-wrist bent, hand raised towards ceiling (picture A). This is now hand A. Using the hand of the uninjured side (hand B), push down on the backside of hand A while hand A resists (hand A is trying to hold it's position). Hold for 3 seconds, do 3 times, do 1 time per day.

A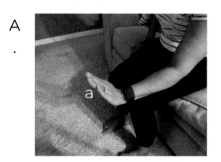

B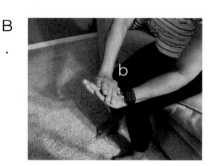

- Isometric radial deviation: Start with arm and hand of the injured side as pictured-wrist bent sideways, hand raised towards celing on thumb side (picture A). This is now hand A. Using the hand of the uninjured side (hand B), push down on the thumbside of hand A while hand A resists (hand A is trying to hold it's position). Hold for 3 seconds, do 3 times, do 1 time per day.

A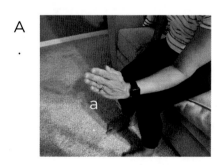

B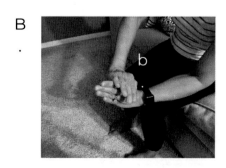

- Isometric ulnar deviation: Start with arm and hand of the injured side as pictured-wrist bent, hand bent down towards ground on pinky side (picture A). This is now hand A. Using the hand of the uninjured side (hand B), push up on the pinky side of hand A while hand A resists (hand A is trying to hold it's position). Hold for 3 seconds, do 3 times, do 1 time per day.

A

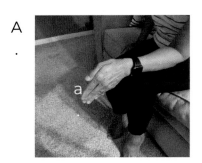

B

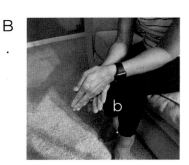

- Eccentric wrist flexion: Start with hand B (of the uninjured side) positioning hand A (of the injured side) into the position shown as in picture A (hand A holding light weight or water bottle, curled up at wrist with hand B holding it in position). Hand B then releases hand A and hand A slowly/with control brings the weight towards the ground (picture B and C). Hand B then repositions hand A (picture A). Do 10 times, 3 sets, 1 time per day.

A

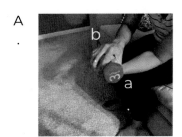

B

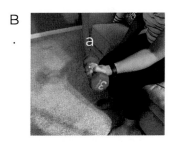

C

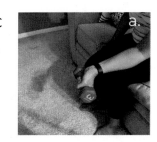

- Eccentric wrist extension: Start with hand B (of the uninjured side) positioning hand A (of the injured side) into the position shown in picture A (hand A holding light weight or water bottle, curled up at wrist with hand B holding it in position). Hand B then releases hand A and hand A slowly and with control brings the weight towards the ground (picture B and C). Hand B then repositions hand A (picture A). Do 10 times, 3 sets, 1 time per day.

A
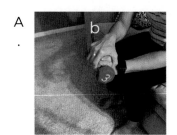

B
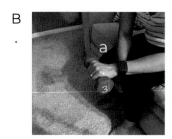

C
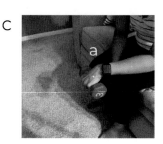

- Eccentric radial deviation: Start with hand B (of the uninjured side) positioning hand A (of the injured side) into the position shown in picture A (hand A holding light weight or water bottle, curled up at wrist on thumbside with hand B holding it in position). Hand B then releases hand A and hand A slowly and with control brings the weight towards the ground (picture B). Hand B then repositions hand A (picture A). Do 10 times, 3 sets, 1 time per day.

A
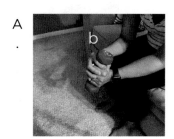

B
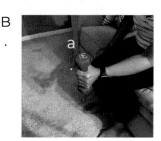

C
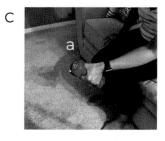

REVIEW

01 We are finally at the week where we can start wrist strengthening! Hurray!

Tasks Completed For Week 7

	M	Tu	W	Th	F	Sa	Su
Wear my brace day and night	○	○	○	○	○	○	○
Kinesiotape	○	○	○	○	○	○	○
Edema glove and massage	○	○	○	○	○	○	○
	○	○	○	○	○	○	○
Soft tissue massage	○	○	○	○	○	○	○
Instrument assisted soft tissue massage	○	○	○	○	○	○	○
Pin and stretch	○	○	○	○	○	○	○
	○	○	○	○	○	○	○
	○	○	○	○	○	○	○
Active Range of Motion Exercises	○	○	○	○	○	○	○
Passive Range of Motion Exercises	○	○	○	○	○	○	○
Upper Body Range of Motion Exercises	○	○	○	○	○	○	○
Become more aware and improve how I am performing	○	○	○	○	○	○	○
my everyday tasks	○	○	○	○	○	○	○

Tasks Completed
For Week 7

	M	Tu	W	Th	F	Sa	Su
Perform exercises for the shoulder girdle	○	○	○	○	○	○	○
Perform exercises for the trunk	○	○	○	○	○	○	○
Perform exercises for the forearm,	○	○	○	○	○	○	○
arm and shoulder	○	○	○	○	○	○	○
Perform exercises for the wrist	○	○	○	○	○	○	○
	○	○	○	○	○	○	○
	○	○	○	○	○	○	○
	○	○	○	○	○	○	○
	○	○	○	○	○	○	○
	○	○	○	○	○	○	○
	○	○	○	○	○	○	○
	○	○	○	○	○	○	○
	○	○	○	○	○	○	○
	○	○	○	○	○	○	○

My dearest friend,

How far you have come!!

We are almost at the finish line! Do you see it?!

How incredible you have been to keep persisting even while life is crazy and demanding.

I am so glad that you continued to put yourself first. Future you is going to thank you.

I applaud you.

Warmly,
Rose

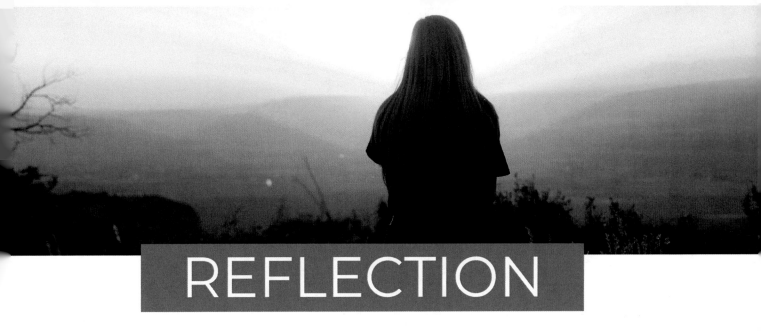

REFLECTION

We are almost there. Almost to the finish line! How do you feel?! Are you ecstatic? Are you in disbelief? Or are you the type (like me) where you don't exactly "feel" anything until you've actually crossed the finish line? If you like, share it with me. I would love to hear about your thoughts!

_____

_____

_____

_____

_____

_____

_____

_____

_____

_____

_____

_____

_____

_____

_____

_____

_____

Week 8

Strengthening The Wrists (Part 2) and The Hands

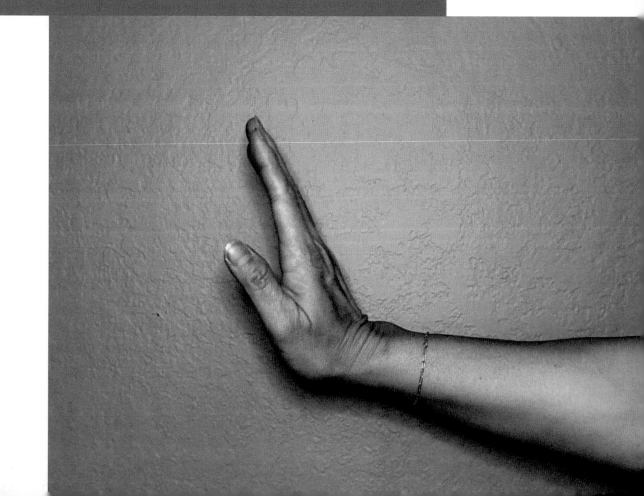

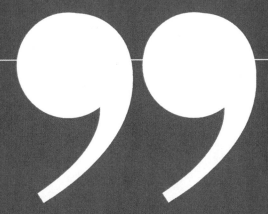

Fall seven times, stand up eight.

JAPANESE PROVERB

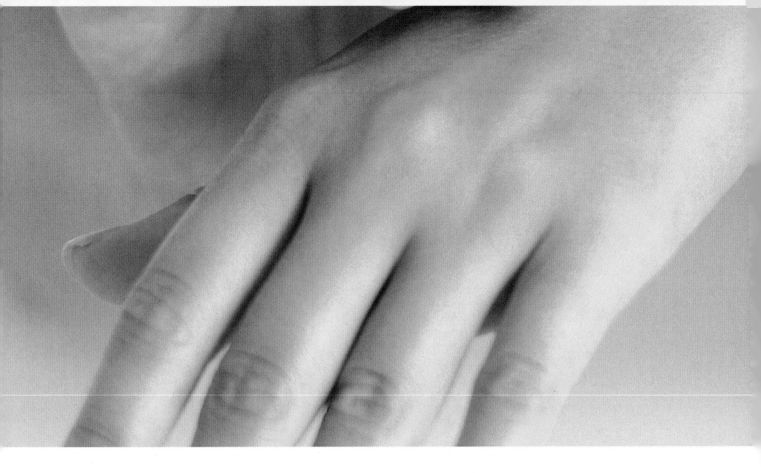

Week 8

Strengthening The Wrists (Part 2) and Hands

Now that we have begun strengthening the wrists, we can go ahead and progress them further and....add strengthening for the hands! FINALLY!!

Tasks To Do This Week

1. Wear a brace at night.

2. Kinesiotape.

3. Wear an edema glove.

4. Perform soft tissue work daily.

5. Range of motion exercises.

Tasks To Do This Week

6. Perform everyday tasks safer to prevent injury and pain to the hands and wrists.

7. Strengthen the shoulder girdle and the trunk.

8. Strengthen the forearm, arm and shoulder.

9. Strengthen the wrist.

10. Strengthen the wrist and hand.

Strengthening The Wrists (Part 2)

Wrist exercises

- Wrist flexion: Start with arm and hand of injured side as pictured (picture A). Then bend your hand up towards the ceiling as pictured (picture B). Return to starting position (picture A). You can either use light weights or a small can/water bottle. Do 2 sets of 10 repetitions, 1 time per day.

A.
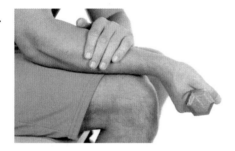

B.
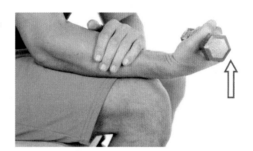

- Wrist extension: Start with arm and hand of injured side as pictured (picture A). Then bend your hand up towards the ceiling as pictured (picture B). Return to starting position (picture A). You can either use light weights or a small can/water bottle. Do 2 sets of 10 repetitions, 1 time per day.

A.
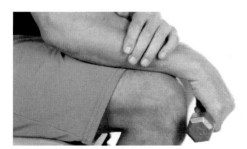

B.
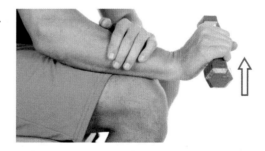

- Radial deviation: Start with arm and hand of injured side as pictured (picture A). Then bend your hand up towards the ceiling as pictured (picture B). Return to starting position (picture A). You can either use light weights or a small can/ water bottle. Do 2 sets of 10 repetitions, 1 time per day.

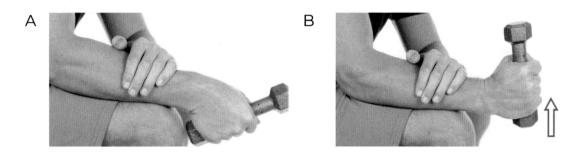

- Ulnar deviation: Start with arm and hand of injured side as pictured (picture A). Then bend your hand up towards the ceiling as pictured (picture B). Return to starting position (picture A). You can either use light weights or a small can/water bottle. Do 2 sets of 10 repetitions, 1 time per day.

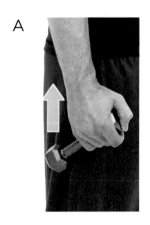
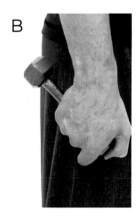

Strengthening The Hands

Hand exercises

- Lumbrical strengthening: Start with your hand of the injured side shaped like the mouth of a duck (see picture A), place towel in between fingers and thumb (see picture B). Squeeze towel by bringing thumb to rest of four fingers (picture C). Return to starting position (picture A). Do 2 sets of 10 repetitions, 1 time per day.

A.

B.

C.

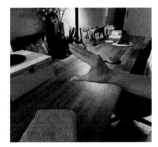 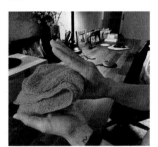 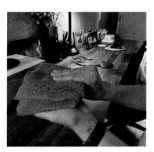

- Grip strengthening: Grip and release a rolled up towel as pictured. Do 2 sets of 10 repetitions, 1 time per day.

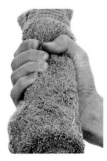

- Finger abduction/adduction: Start by placing a towel on a table. Place hand of injured side flat on the towel (picture A). Slide your fingers together tightly (picture B). Spread your fingers apart as wide as possible (picture C). Alternate between picture B and C until you have done 2 sets of 10 repetitions, 1 time per day.

A 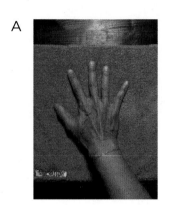 B 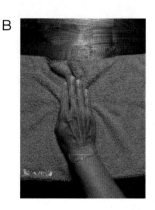 C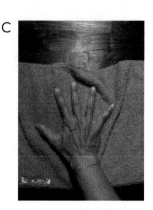

- Thumb adduction: Start by gripping a towel with the index, middle, ring and small finger of the injured side(picture A). Press your thumb into the side of the index finger and towel (picture B). Relax and return to starting position (picture A). Do 2 sets of 10 repetitions, 1 time per day.

A 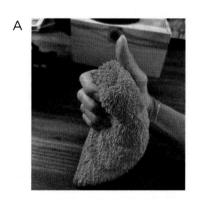 B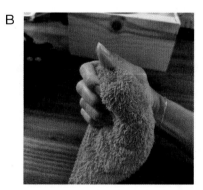

- Finger open/close: Placing a rubber band around all five fingers of the injured hand, open the hand (picture A) and then close the hand (picture B). Repeat. Do 2 sets of 10, 1 time per day.

A 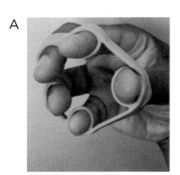   B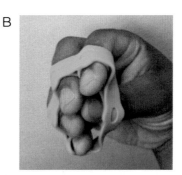

- Thumb abduction: Start by placing a rubber band around all fingers of the injured hand as picture A and B shows. Stretch out your thumb as picture C shows. Relax and return to starting position (picture B). Do 2 sets of 10 repetitions, 1 time per day.

A 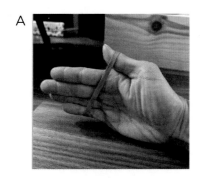   B 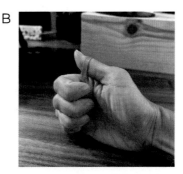   C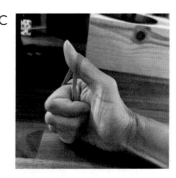

REVIEW

01   Continue progressing your wrist strengthening.   Yay we can start hand strengthening!

Tasks Completed For Week 8

	M	Tu	W	Th	F	Sa	Su
Wear my brace day and night	◯	◯	◯	◯	◯	◯	◯
Kinesiotape	◯	◯	◯	◯	◯	◯	◯
Edema glove and massage	◯	◯	◯	◯	◯	◯	◯
	◯	◯	◯	◯	◯	◯	◯
Soft tissue massage	◯	◯	◯	◯	◯	◯	◯
Instrument assisted soft tissue massage	◯	◯	◯	◯	◯	◯	◯
Pin and stretch	◯	◯	◯	◯	◯	◯	◯
	◯	◯	◯	◯	◯	◯	◯
	◯	◯	◯	◯	◯	◯	◯
Active Range of Motion Exercises	◯	◯	◯	◯	◯	◯	◯
Passive Range of Motion Exercises	◯	◯	◯	◯	◯	◯	◯
Upper Body Range of Motion Exercises	◯	◯	◯	◯	◯	◯	◯
Become more aware and improve how I am performing my everyday tasks	◯	◯	◯	◯	◯	◯	◯
	◯	◯	◯	◯	◯	◯	◯

Tasks Completed
For Week 8

	M	Tu	W	Th	F	Sa	Su
Perform exercises for the shoulder girdle	○	○	○	○	○	○	○
Perform exercises for the trunk	○	○	○	○	○	○	○
Perform exercises for the forearm,	○	○	○	○	○	○	○
arm and shoulder	○	○	○	○	○	○	○
Perform exercises for the wrist	○	○	○	○	○	○	○
Perform exercises for the hand	○	○	○	○	○	○	○
	○	○	○	○	○	○	○
	○	○	○	○	○	○	○
	○	○	○	○	○	○	○
	○	○	○	○	○	○	○
	○	○	○	○	○	○	○
	○	○	○	○	○	○	○
	○	○	○	○	○	○	○
	○	○	○	○	○	○	○

You did it!!!

You came, you persevered and

YOU CONQUERED!!

I am so proud of what you have achieved,
but I am even more proud that you showed up.

Every day.

Because that takes strength and bravery.

I hope you are feeling quite proud of yourself too.

I wish I could be there in person to give you a hug, but
here's one in spirit.

YOU ARE MY HERO!

Warmly,
Rose

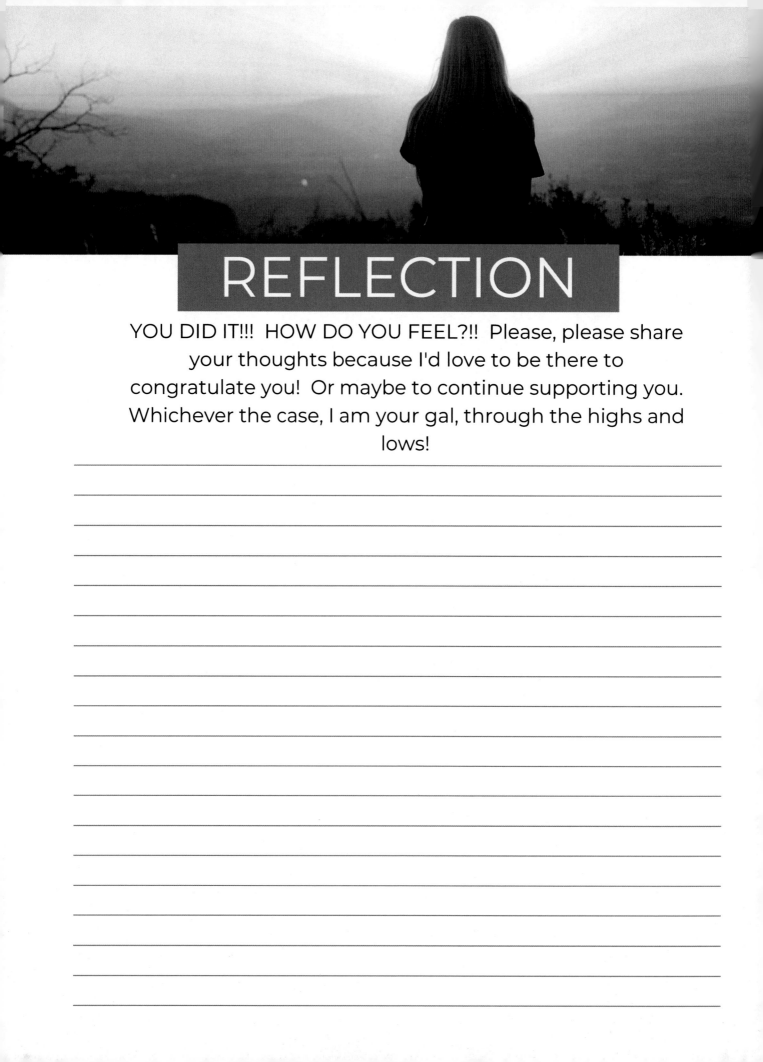

REFLECTION

YOU DID IT!!! HOW DO YOU FEEL?!! Please, please share your thoughts because I'd love to be there to congratulate you! Or maybe to continue supporting you. Whichever the case, I am your gal, through the highs and lows!

_____
_____
_____
_____
_____
_____
_____
_____
_____
_____
_____
_____
_____
_____
_____
_____
_____

Oh my, oh my, oh my!! I could not be more proud of you than I am right now!!

A few last instructions before I send you back to your life with much less pain!

1. You can completely stop wearing your brace. I know it will feel a little nerve wracking at first and you might feel little twinges of pain and stiffness, but you are ready. If you start to feel a slight increase in pain, then go back to wearing it at night for another week. After that week try again to discontinue brace wear.

2. You can also discontinue kinesiotaping and edema glove wear.

3. Continue all your soft tissue work and exercises daily for another 2-3 weeks. After that I would recommend doing these exercises 1-2 times per week for life.

4. Continue all that you've learned about safe performance of your daily activities. These teachings should be a permanent part of your life!

EQUIPMENT I RECOMMEND
(Click on links)

For cellphone use

1. Cellphone cover
2. Cellphone holder: for example, a <u>ring</u> or <u>popsocket</u>

For childcare

1. A nursing pillow: for example the <u>My Brest Friend nursing pillow</u>
2. A hip seat carrier: for example the <u>Tush Baby</u>
3. <u>A baby carrier</u>

For the kitchen

1. <u>Jar gripper</u> to open items
2. <u>Cooking tools and utensils with bigger handles</u>
3. <u>Palm brush</u> to wash dishes (not a scrub wand)

EQUIPMENT I RECOMMEND
(Click on links)

For work

1. <u>Pens with a larger diameter</u>
2. Ergonomic mouse: for example a <u>vertical mouse</u>
3. Ergonomic keyboard: for example a <u>split keyboard</u>
4. Ergonomic scissors: for example a <u>spring loaded one</u>

kinesiotape

1. KT tape pro extreme---><u>click here for link</u>

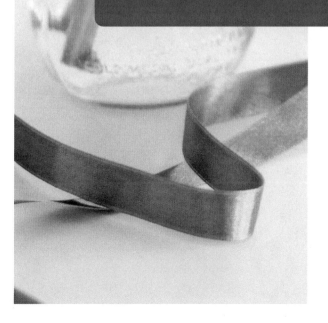

General Tips To Take Care Of Your Hands and Wrists

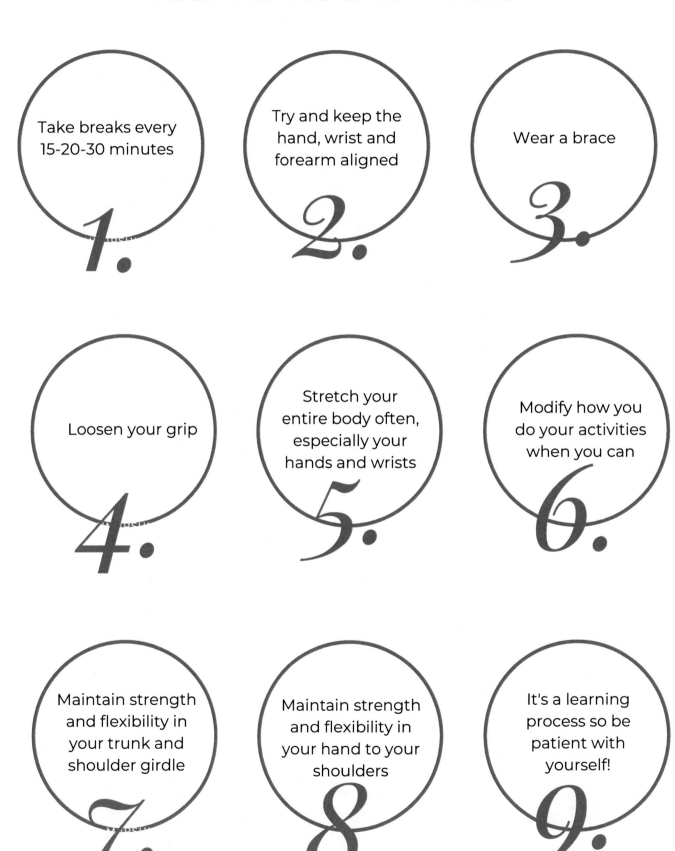

Take breaks every 15-20-30 minutes

1.

Try and keep the hand, wrist and forearm aligned

2.

Wear a brace

3.

Loosen your grip

4.

Stretch your entire body often, especially your hands and wrists

5.

Modify how you do your activities when you can

6.

Maintain strength and flexibility in your trunk and shoulder girdle

7.

Maintain strength and flexibility in your hand to your shoulders

8.

It's a learning process so be patient with yourself!

9.

Taking care of your hands and wrists start with
taking care of yourself

What is one main goal that you will try to start incorporating into your life? It can be big or small.

Break up the main goal into smaller monthly self-care tasks:

☐ _____   ☐ _____

☐ _____   ☐ _____

☐ _____   ☐ _____

☐ _____   ☐ _____

☐ _____   ☐ _____

☐ _____   ☐ _____

Which tasks have been your favorite that you can keep doing permanently?

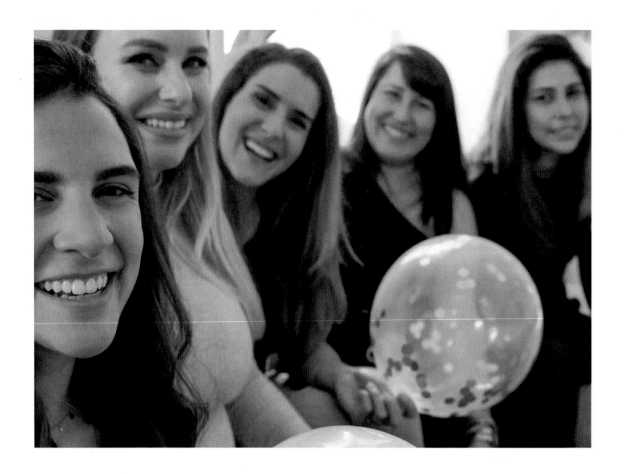

Congratulations!!

A huge congratulations to you!! You've done it! You have completed this guide!!
I am so proud of the dedication you put in to learn how to care for your hand and wrist pain. It is a huge endeavor and you didn't shy away. That takes so much strength from deep within.

I have faith in you that you will continue to keep yourself well, but if you need anything I'm not far away. Don't hesitate to reach out.

Again, CONGRATULATIONS!!

With love, Rose

First The MOMS

IF YOU WOULD LIKE MORE IN DEPTH GUIDANCE

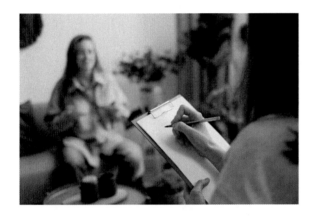 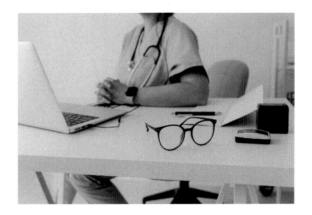

We offer the opportunity to work with our expert Rose one-on-one. With that we can look more in depth into your injury and provide a personalized program. This allows for more success!

We also offer other various products and services to help in your recovery!

CLICK HERE TO LEARN MORE:

YES, I'D LIKE TO WORK WITH ROSE

OR CLICK BELOW TO GO TO OUR WEBSITE
OR INSTAGRAM:

WWW.FIRSTTHEMOMS.COM

@FIRSTTHEMOMS

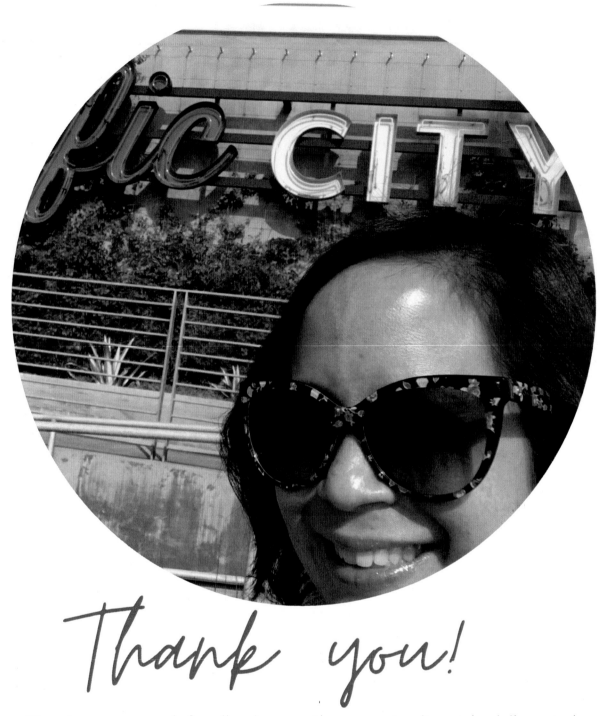

Thank you!

Thank you so much for allowing me the opportunity and privilege to be a part of your recovery! It is my passion and my joy to be able to help Moms in this way.

Please don't hesitage to contact me if you need any further support, help or guidance!

Rose

Made in the USA
Las Vegas, NV
23 April 2024

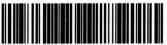

89044923R00102